C

4406.

To do the sick no harm

International Library of Social Policy

General Editor   Kathleen Jones
Professor of Social Administration
University of York

Arbor Scientiæ
Arbor Vitæ

A catalogue of the books available in the **International Library
of Social Policy** and other series of Social Science books published
by Routledge & Kegan Paul will be found at the end of this volume

To do the sick no harm

A study of the British voluntary hospital system to 1875

John Woodward

Department of Economic History
University of Sheffield

Routledge & Kegan Paul

London and Boston

First published in 1974
by Routledge & Kegan Paul Ltd
Broadway House, 68–74 Carter Lane,
London EC4V 5EL and
9 Park Street,
Boston, Mass. 02108, USA
Set in Monotype Times New Roman
and printed in Great Britain by
Unwin Brothers Limited
The Gresham Press
Old Woking, Surrey
© John Woodward 1974
No part of this book may be reproduced in
any form without permission from the
publisher, except for the quotation of brief
passages in criticism

ISBN 0 7100 7970 2
Library of Congress Catalog Card No. 74–81999

To my parents

Contents

Acknowledgments

I am indebted to the Health Research Unit of the Institute of Social and Economic Research in the University of York which originally provided the finance for this study and gave me excellent working facilities. The authorities of the hospitals concerned were extremely co-operative in allowing me access to their records and I wish to thank them for their generous assistance. My thanks are due to the library staff of the Wellcome Institute of the History of Medicine, without whose unfailing assistance no work of this kind could be completed; they answered my innumerable queries with great patience over a number of years. The editor of the *Royal College of General Practitioners, Yorkshire Faculty Journal*, has allowed me to use material which originally appeared in the autumn 1969 issue in an article entitled 'Before bacteriology, deaths in hospitals'. My typist, Mrs Helen Cox, has coped with me as an anxious author and with my untidy script with little apparent signs of strain. I must thank three members of staff in the University of York: Edmund Cooney provided much constructive criticism; Professor Eric Sigsworth gave me the initial impetus to tackle this subject as a doctoral thesis and acted as my supervisor with all the problems that this duty involves; and finally the editor of this series Professor Kathleen Jones. Despite all these people to whom I owe thanks, the errors and omissions which remain are solely my responsibility.

Introduction

The writing of any type of history is fraught with difficulties. The historian is concerned always about the nature of the data available and about the interpretation which can be derived from the evidence, and yet it is not easy to define the boundaries of historical study as a whole for the areas of study constantly change and expand. Recently, there has been considerable interest in expanding these boundaries by developing a number of specialist branches of history, ranging from industrial archaeology to urban history. Each of these new areas of research has added new facets to our knowledge of the past, and the history of medicine, to which this book is a contribution, has yet another dimension to offer. The history of medicine in all its forms, from the development of drug therapy to the impact of medical changes on society, is one of the legitimate fields of research interest but it is one which has been strangely neglected by historians.

The comparative lack of interest in the subject stems, perhaps, from the mystique which surrounds medical science. Members of the medical profession are held with some regard by the majority of people and the medical terminology involved is a considerable barrier to an understanding of the subject. There have been many major studies in the history of medicine, principally undertaken by medically qualified authors, but their contributions are not widely known or understood by historians.

Yet, there is much to be gained by co-operation between the historian of medicine and the general historian in understanding the impact of medical phenomena on economies and on society. The possibility of such fruitful co-operation has been shown in two recent collections of essays (G. McLachlan and T. McKeown (eds), *Medical History and Medical Care*, 1971; and E. Clarke (ed.), *Modern Methods in the History of Medicine*, 1973). These works indicate the mutual benefit to be gained from relating various aspects of the social and applied sciences to the history of medicine, and the history of medicine to other aspects of history and to present-day problems in medical practice.

This present book attempts to answer a problem which has not previously been examined fully because of the difficulties of entering the history of medicine by, in particular, economic and social historians. The study is concerned principally with the contribution of the general voluntary hospitals in Britain to the health of the population during the eighteenth and nineteenth centuries. Many histories of individual hospitals have been written but, with a few notable exceptions, they have been concerned solely with the finance and the administration of the institution under consideration; while little attention has been paid to the work of the hospitals with regard to the patients.

Initially, an examination is made of the provision of medical treatment available to the population until the upswelling of a philanthropic movement to establish voluntary hospitals (and dispensaries) in the early eighteenth century catering for the working poor of the country. Administrative and staffing procedures are studied as a preliminary to looking at the patients and their problems. Three major influences on the chances of survival in the hospitals are analysed in detail: the admissions policy with regard to fever patients, the number and nature of surgical operations, and the incidence of sepsis. The purpose is to attempt a reply to the statement made by Professor B. Abel-Smith that: 'Hardly anything is said about the effects which developments in hospital services have had on mortality inside and outside the hospital . . . facts are far too few. . . . Detailed analysis of the case records of individual hospitals, allied to other systematic studies, would be needed before any conclusions could be reached about mortality or morbidity' (*The Hospitals 1800–1948*, p. 10).

Thus, this book attempts to bring together a number of different types of history, from the political and economic motives behind eighteenth-century philanthropy to the effectiveness of improvements in medical facilities and treatment. It is a partial study in bridging the gap between traditional historians and medical historians. Perhaps, with more, and better, works of this kind the history of medicine will be accepted as a subject worthy of further exploration not only as a subject in itself, but also as a contribution to a better understanding of our past.

1   Medical care and social policy

In A.D. 947 the canons of York Minister founded the Hospital of St Peter, the earliest authenticated hospital in Great Britain. This hospital was designed probably as a hostel for the traveller or pilgrim rather than as an institution for the care of the sick, as were the many other similar institutions which followed. In later years the hospitals began to employ physicians and to care for the sick, for disease was thought to be the result of God's will and so its treatment fell upon the members of the church. As treatment consisted mainly of rest, diet and the dressing of sores, the clergy were well able to undertake this task. From the time of the Norman Conquest hospitals were established in all parts of the country, either by religious orders or by the monarch or by other wealthy persons who were connected with the church. Thus, the concept of a hospital took on a dual role – that of a hostel and that of an institution for the care of the sick. A religious hospital:[1]

> was an ecclesiastical, not a medical, institution. It was for care rather than for cure: for the relief of the body, when possible, but pre-eminently for the refreshment of the soul. By manifold religious observances, the staff sought to elevate and discipline character. They endeavoured, as the body decayed, to strengthen the soul and prepare it for the future life. Faith and love were more predominant features in hospital life than were skill and science.

The first institution founded to fulfil the practice of a hospital as we know it today was St Bartholomew's in London, established by Rahere in 1123. It gave help to the needy and poor of the district, including orphans and outcasts, and provided relief to every kind of sick person and wayfarer. The sick poor were treated until they recovered, and if a mother died in the hospital her child was to be cared for until the age of seven. Other hospitals continued to be founded and endowed until the onset of the Reformation, including that of St Thomas's.[2]

However, abuses crept into the system and the larger monasteries

1

began to remove their hospitals or allowed them to fall into decay. Henry VIII promised Parliament that if the religious houses were handed over to his care the poor and the sick would not suffer, and as a result their dissolution was put into effect with little or no public outcry, the smaller houses in 1536 and the larger ones in 1539.

In 1538 the mayor, aldermen and commonalty of the City of London petitioned the king to refound a number of the religious houses. They considered that the houses for the care of the sick poor were not like the other houses 'for the maintenance of priests, canons, and clerks living carnally as they had done lately, nothing regarding the miserable people living in the street, offending every clean person passing by the way with their filthy and nasty savors'.[3] As a result of this petition five royal or chartered hospitals were established by the end of the sixteenth century.[4] From this time until the foundation of the voluntary hospitals in the eighteenth century, these five institutions were the only hospitals available to the sick poor – a lamentably small number.[5]

The state of medical provision for the mass of the population was put in a vivid form by Samuel Garth, the poet-physician, when he gave an oration to his colleagues of the College of Physicians of London at the end of the seventeenth century:[6]

> But at present. . . . Medicine itself is sick. This Art, of all others
> the most useful, knows not how to help itself; while rather
> from mock Physicians, than diseases, this country suffers. What,
> and what sort of people they are, the rubrick'd walls at the
> corner of every street will inform you. Here an operator,
> mounted on his pyed horse, draws teeth in the streets; another
> is so obliging, as to be at home at certain hours to receive
> fools; another pores in urinals, and if he finds no disease there,
> he makes it; another still, draws together a crowd by the help
> of rope-dancing; he comes, he sees, then rushes forth upon the
> multitude and murders without mercy. Yet not with weapons do
> these swarms of mountebanks inflict wounds, but with some
> nostrums more dangerous than any weapon.

Medical facilities were completely unorganized and virtually uncontrolled, except in the immediate vicinity of London. For the wealthy medical treatment was available from the physicians and surgeons, but for the poor this was not possible. A report of 1690 suggested that 'The usual Fee of a Doctor in ancient times was 20s. and that had not taken that Degree, 10s. But now there is no certain

Rule, but some that are Eminent have received in Fees Yearly 2000 or 3000£'.[7] At this time approximately one-fifth of the total population was earning probably less than £7 a year. John Radcliffe (1650–1714), the physician,[8] received no less than 600 guineas a year alone from William III for royal consultations, and he passed on many of his patients to Richard Mead (1673–1754), who, it is estimated, earned between £5,000 and £6,000 yearly. These were, naturally, the most eminent members of their profession, but the fees and salaries indicate that their services were out of the reach of the ordinary man. The same was true of surgeons who normally performed operations in the patient's home. It was only in the case of serious illness that a physician or surgeon would be approached and then only when an agreement was reached to waive or reduce the usual fee.[9]

Beneath the physicians and surgeons in status were the apothecaries who were allowed to charge for their medicines but not for their advice. Those who could not afford the fees of the physicians and surgeons turned to the apothecaries for treatment, who could be described as tradesmen rather than craftsmen, being generally qualified only in the art of medicine.

The demands of all classes were met by the quacks who were plentiful not only in this country, but also on the Continent. It has been estimated that in the county of Lincoln alone the quacks outnumbered registered practitioners by nine to one in 1804,[10] although the most successful era for quacks was the eighteenth century. As Garth suggested, many of the quacks were utter charlatans, but it should be remembered that several were very skilful men.[11] Certainly there were many charlatans who deceived the public, but if their remedies were harmless placebos little damage could be done; the quacks kept the people content while the illness was being cured by the natural workings of the body.

Probably the main provision for the sick poor came from within the family itself: 'A folklore or quasi-medical knowledge was handed down from mother to daughter and no doubt the advice of neighbours, friends and priests was taken if not always used.'[12] Little positive action could be taken as the idea that illness was an affliction from God still prevailed. A number of publications were available to the lay reader on medical matters, the most notable being William Buchan's *Domestic Medicine* which went through several editions during the eighteenth and early nineteenth centuries.

Paupers, as distinct from the poor, had access to medical treatment by virtue of the section of the Elizabethan Poor Law of 1601 which ordered the parish to provide 'necessary relief of the lame, impotent, old, blind, and such other among them . . . not able to work'.[13] Some authorities employed the local surgeon or apothecary to treat the paupers, at a salary of £12 to £20 yearly, though from this sum the practitioner had to meet the cost of the medicines. However, their numbers were few as many of the parish authorities could not afford to pay the necessary salary and even after the Act permitting parishes to provide joint workhouses the numbers were small. In 1732, seven years after the passing of the Act, there were only 115 workhouses in Great Britain, fifty of which were in London, and only one in Scotland, situated in Glasgow. The parish authorities in London, working together through the Common Council, paid for the treatment of patients at the chartered hospitals, but the problem was complicated as many of the inhabitants were not living in the parish of their birth and therefore were not eligible for relief. Thus, the medical facilities provided by the parish authorities varied from area to area and were virtually non-existent in many.

It is against this background of totally inadequate medical provision for the bulk of the population that at the end of the seventeenth century the College of Physicians of London attempted to found a dispensary, but because of the animosity raging between the College and the Society of Apothecaries it was of no avail. In 1687 the College requested its fellows, candidates and licentiates to give advice, free of charge, to the poor in the City and in the surrounding seven miles where their monopoly extended. It was suggested that by providing such a service the physicians would both recommend themselves to the public and enhance their own knowledge and reputation for success. Ten years later, in April 1697, the College opened a dispensary without the co-operation of the Society of Apothecaries:[14]

The members of the College of Physicians have collected (by way of a Charitable Subscription) a Joynt-stock of about 500 l. to prepare at the said College all sorts of Medicines for the Poor, and to give them at intrinsick Value, that is, for what they only cost, which will save the Poor 15 s. in the Pound; the Physicians have likewise obligated themselves voluntarily, under a forfeiture, to attend the College in turns, to give Advice to all People that will come thither for nothing, every Wednesday and Saturday in the Afternoon, all the year.

The London Dispensary for Sick-Poor, as it was known, came constantly under attack from the Society of Apothecaries, but it appears that in 1701 the Society voted that they 'should offer the Corporation for setting the poore on Worke to furnish them gratis with necessary medicines for three Years'.[15] The Dispensary continued to function until 1725 when the College decided not to lease out the rooms then in use as the Dispensary, but no reasons are given for its discontinuance. In Scotland, a dispensary had been founded in 1682 by the College of Physicians of Edinburgh to provide medical treatment for the sick poor of the city and the surrounding area, but it was organized on a purely informal basis.

Although these two dispensaries provided much-needed medical attention, they were too few and could not give adequate care to the patients who required constant attention or specialized treatment.[16]

B

2   To prove a need

Outside the few work-house infirmaries, no public accommodation was then available for the sick poor except the two chartered hospitals, which had become quite inadequate at a peculiarly distressful period to the needs of the then population. The imposition at those institutions of a demand for fees from all applicants for admission acted as a class limitation by excluding those in direct need, who were unable to procure the necessary money, yet were ineligible from one cause or another for parish relief. For them no alternative was left but unrelieved suffering, yet they were the very persons for whom the chartered hospitals were originally intended.[1]

Despite the lack of medical facilities in Great Britain at the beginning of the eighteenth century the idea of public provision was a very old one. In St Thomas More's *Utopia* (1516):[2]

Special care is taken of the sick who are looked after in public hospitals. They have four at the city limits, a little outside the walls. These are so roomy as to be comparable to as many small towns. The purpose is twofold: first, that the sick, however numerous, should not be packed too close together in consequent discomfort and, second, that those who have a contagious disease likely to pass from one to another may be isolated as much as possible from the rest.

In the seventeenth century a similar work on social and economic reforms featured a 'College of Experience, where they deliver out, yearly, such medicines as they find out by experience; and all such as shall be able to demonstrate any experiment, for the health or wealth of other men, are honourably rewarded at the publick charge'.[3] As a direct result of this book a pamphlet appeared from William Petty, advocating, among many other reforms, a fully equipped hospital where disease could be investigated.[4] 'A true lover of this country' suggested in 1667 that a hospital for foundlings and for pregnant women should be founded; he further recommended a system of direct payments to medical practitioners to provide free advice and medicines to all sick or wounded people 'allowed in forma pauperis to require their assistance'.[5] Later in the century Hugh Chamberlen (the man-midwife) proposed that all sick people should be eligible for medical attention. The scheme would be financed by an assessment of every house, excepting charity cases, and he estimated that 7 hospitals would be required in London, staffed by 164 physicians, 121 surgeons and 149 apothecaries.[6]

Towards the end of the seventeenth century it was William Petty who was to influence the framework within which the health of the country was considered. Health, according to a lecture he delivered in 1676, was the keystone to prosperity:[7]

Now suppose that in the King's Dominions there be 9 millions of people, of which 360,000 dye every year, and from whom 440,000 are borne. And suppose that by the advancement of the art of Medicine, a quarter part fewer dye. Then the King will gain and save 200,000 subjects per annum, which valued at 20£ per head, the lowest price of slaves, will make 4 million per annum benefit to the Commonwealth.

He repeated his demand for hospitals in the same lecture and commented that:[8]

Another cause of defect in the art of medicine and consequently of its contempt is that there have not been Hospitalls for the Accommodation of sick people. Rich as well as Poor, so instituted and fitted as to encourage all sick persons to resort unto them – Every sort of such hospitalls to differ only in splendor, but not at all in the Sufficiency for the means and remedy for the Patients health. For by such means the most able understandings might be encouraged, equally with the best of the professions, to spend and dedicate themselves to this faculty; and a man shall learn in a well regulated hospitall, where he may within halfe a hower's time observe his choice of 1000 patients, more in one yeare then in ten without it, even by reading the best Books that can be written.

A contemporary of Petty, Nehemiah Grew, a physician, adopted many of Petty's ideas in a pamphlet he produced for Queen Anne in 1707. He considered that prosperity was dependent on the size of the population and that the government should do all in its power to control health. As the sick cost the state more than the dead he proposed that physicians' fees should be regulated, according to experience, so that the cost of medical care could be reduced and thus become readily available to all.[9]

However, all these ideas did not produce any immediately tangible results. The proposals needed a well-developed local administration working under strong central supervision, but, towards the end of the seventeenth century, it was exactly this type of control which was being allowed to lapse. For a period of five hundred years neither the church nor the state chose to help the sick by founding hospitals. 'There is no really satisfying explanation. It has been suggested that perhaps the new medical profession frowned upon the hospitals and preferred to keep such surgery as was undertaken in its own hands. But the explanation does not ring true.'[10] Certainly the climate of opinion, as judged by the publications of the day, did not concern itself overwhelmingly with health. Even the works considered here were concerned primarily with the economic rather than the social aspects of the health of the labouring poor.

The beginning of the eighteenth century saw the re-awakening of a philanthropic frame of mind; Queen Anne's death in 1714 heralded the end of the Act of Schism and a new religious liberty took its place. 'Latitudinarianism once again became the order of the day, and the principles of a truer religion inculcating charity and toleration were fostered by the Low Church party and the Nonconformists.'[11] It was also a time of unprecedented wealth for the few after the War of the Spanish Succession and the Treaty of Utrecht which followed. There was the example of the continental hospitals which had not been dissolved at the time of the Reformation, the Hôtel Dieu in Paris stood witness to the traditional values of Catholicism and the former Catholic institutions in the Netherlands flourished under the Protestants. 'The example of the Dutch found a ready welcome among low churchmen and dissenters intent upon good works.'[12] In Great Britain for one small part of the population, poor French Protestants, M. de Gastigny (once Master of the Buckhounds to the Prince of Orange), bequeathed £1,000 for a hospital on his death in 1708. It was opened in London, as a hospice, in 1716 with accommodation for eighty people. The institution probably admitted the sick as the sixteenth rule stated that the house visitors had to make inquiries 'whether among the Poor, there may be not some who having been taken into the Hospital as sick in body and Disordered in Mind, are so well recovered as to be fit to be discharged'.[13] Though this hospital served a small minority of the population, and differed from the eventual structure of the voluntary hospitals in that it paid its medical staff, it probably acted as an example to the rest of the community.

John Bellers, a Quaker, put the new feelings of the people into print in his famous twelve proposals.[14] In this essay (1714), having made a study of the hospitals in the Netherlands, he urged the erection of hospitals and the provision of adequate medical treatment for the sick poor. The first half of the work, following from the calculations of William Petty, is an attempt to give some value to the cost of ill-health. He computes that 200,000 people die annually in Great Britain and 'that a Hundred Thousand, of those Two Hundred Thousand, Die Yearly of Curable Diseases; for want of Timely Advice, and Suitable Medicines'.[15] He continues:[16]

> Considering that above Three Quarters of our People are Poor, and not able to procure either, but what's of CHARITY; and therefore many of them must be Lost, and Die Miserably, for want of a suitable Provision for them. . . . And if the other part of our People can procure a Physician's Attendance, yet Diseases and Medicines are so Mysterious in many Cases, and of those which are known by some Physicians, are but little understood by many others, that it may be questioned, whether one Half of the Rich may not Die of such Maladies as would be Curable if Diseases and Medicines were better Understood, and more Universal.

At this point the emphasis of the essay changes to an examination of the productivity of labour and the costs to the nobility and gentry of having their labour force ill or dying. Bellers calculates that one million people are sick annually and that the cost of 'Every Able Industrious Labourer, that is capably to have Children, who so Untimely Dies, may be accounted Two Hundred Pounds Loss to the Kingdom. As for our Nobility and Gentry, I leave their Valuation to themselves.'[17] He pleads for state intervention in medical research and the spreading abroad of medical knowledge by arguing that 'considering the present Deficiency in the Art of Healing, in many Cases; it makes the Improvement of Medicine of the greater Import to all Degrees of People, from the Greatest MONARCH, to the Meanest Peasant'.[18] The conclusion of this section of the essay is a plea to all: 'Wherefore, it's as much the Duty of the Poor to Labour when

they are Able, as it is for the Rich to Help them when they are
Sick'.[19]

The second half of the essay is taken up with the twelve proposals
to improve the general medical provision of Great Britain. They are
enumerated in the following manner:[20]

> (1) THAT there should be Built, at, or near London, HOSPITALS
> for the POOR; if not one HOSPITAL for every Particular Capital
> DISTEMPER; for the entertaining of such Poor Patients, whose
> Conditions may Want it; And to have Physicians and
> Chirurgeons suitable to take Care of the SICK. [The knowledge
> gained from this practice was to be made known to all the
> medical profession.]
> (2) That one Hospital should be more particularly under the
> Care and Direction of the QUEEN's Physicians; that they may
> take into it such Patients whose Infirmities at any time, our
> SOVEREIGN may be subject to. . . . [Proposals 3 and 4 recommend
> a hospital for the blind and another for the incurable.]
> (5) That a Publick Laboratory, and a Physical Observatory be
> Provided. . . . [These were to provide medicines and to look for
> new preparations.]
> (6) That there be One Hospital at least, at each of our Two
> UNIVERSITIES. . . .
> (7) That in every Hundred of a County, and Parish of a City,
> there be appointed one Doctor and Chirurgeon (or more; if
> needful) to take Care of the Sick Poor in them; who should
> visit every Parish once a Week, at least. [These practitioners
> were to be paid by the Overseers of the poor.]

The final four proposals are concerned with the discovery and
propagation of knowledge, the important part being:

> (10) That the COLLEGE OF PHYSICIANS, and COMPANY of
> CHIRURGEONS, should draw up a Summary of Advice, in both
> their Faculties, in the plainest manner, of what common Errors
> should be avoided in Practice, as well as what is fit to be done;
> for a general Information to all the Practitioners in PHYSICK and
> CHIRURGERY through the Nation, that they be more successful
> to their Patients.

It has been necessary to give Bellers's proposals in some detail as
his views on hospitals were part of a much larger scheme to remedy
the general lack of medical provision for the bulk of the population.

Although his overall plan was not taken up, as it needed both central and local control, it inspired a number of private individuals to consider a local means of alleviating the sick poor. The first fruits of the scheme can be seen in the preamble to the Westminster Society which was established in January 1716:[21]

> Notwithstanding the provision settled by our laws and the collections made by the charity of well-disposed Christians for the relief of the poor, it is obvious to anyone that walks the streets that the same is not sufficient to preserve great numbers of them from begging to the great grief of all good men, and the no small reproach of our religion and country, etc.
> Frequent attempts have been made to provide for the poor, but hitherto they have been ineffectual; they must depend upon the voluntary assistance of charitable people and a Christian spirit on the part of those persons employed to take care of the poor, etc.

The intention of the charity was to provide a comprehensive service for the sick and pregnant women. Food and physic, the advice of physicians and surgeons and the help of nurses for the sick; and necessary lodging and attendance for pregnant women would be given. Sick prisoners were to be visited and relieved; the destitute were to be given money; and the clergy were to be available to save the souls of the outcasts. It was intended to establish branches in all parts of the city, but this did not come to fruition. Perhaps the aims of the Society were too ambitious, for in three months the benefits had to be limited to the poor living in the parish of St Margaret's and shortly after the complete programme had to be abandoned for lack of funds.

Henry Hoare, the 'good Henry', a banker, who was instrumental in initiating the Westminster Society, tried again, in 1719, to found a charitable institution – an infirmary:[22]

> WHEREAS great Numbers of sick Persons in this City languish for want of Necessaries, and too often die miserably, who are not entitled to a Parochial Relief: And whereas amongst those who do receive Relief from their respective Parishes, many suffer extremely, and are sometimes lost, partly for want of Accommodations and proper Medicines in their own Houses or Lodgings, (the Closeness and Unwholesomeness of which is too often one great Cause of their Sickness) partly by the imprudent

laying out of what is so allowed, and by the Ignorance and
Carelessness or ill Management of those about them. . . .
WE, whose Names are underwritten, in Obedience to the Rules
of our holy Religion, desiring, so far as in us lies, to find some
Remedy for this great Misery of our poor Neighbours do
subscribe the following Sums of Money to be by us paid Yearly
(during Pleasure) by Quarterly Payments, for the procuring,
furnishing, and defraying the necessary Expences of an
Infirmary, or Place of Entertainment, for such poor sick
Persons inhabiting in the Parish of St Margaret, Westminster,
or others, who shall be recommended by any of the
Subscribers or Benefactors, with the Approbation and Consent
of the major Part of the Trustees present; who likewise are
empowered to allow suitable Relief to such sick Persons,
approved in the Manner above mentioned, as are incapable of
being removed from their respective Abodes.

The proposals for the infirmary were very similar to those for the
charitable society with the addition of accommodation for the sick
poor, free of all expense.

The Westminster Infirmary was the first of a new form of charity –
the voluntary hospital. Voluntary hospitals differed from the
chartered institutions in several important respects. They were
dependent on voluntary subscriptions or contributions rather than on
endowments for financial support; subscribers rather than a President
and Governors appointed by charter took care of the administration;
medical and surgical staff held honorary positions, receiving no
salary but usually having the rights of subscribers; and the final
difference was the fact that patients were not required to pay fees.[23]

In the provinces the first voluntary hospital to be founded was
at Winchester. Dr Alured Clarke, prebend of the cathedral since
1723, organized the promotion of this undertaking in what was a
small market town. Clarke put forward the proposal on 22 May
1736, by 6 August the subscription papers were ready for distribution
and on 18 October the first patient was admitted, although the
contributions were £600 short of the target. Despite this generally
favourable response there were a number of objections to the scheme
which had to be countered:[24]

1. It was said that a workhouse is more wanted than a
hospital. It may be enough to observe that whenever a better
provision is made for the sick poor by Parliament this house

will either cease or become part of that provision. The design
now in hand of erecting public workhouses in every county is a
strong argument in favour of the present scheme.

2. It was objected that the poor dislike anything with the
appearance of constraint or removal from their families. But
any who desire it shall be considered and received as out-
patients. Experience tells that whenever a hospital has been
erected the poor have esteemed it a blessing and have flocked
to it with eagerness; for there they get free air, wholesome and
proper diet, clean and constant attendance, the best advice, and
no more medicines than are necessary.

3. Others supposed that a hospital would occasion the resort
of poor people to the city. But no person will be entitled to
receive any medicine unless recommended by a contributor,
and anyone, not inhabiting the city or suburbs, who asks for
alms may be incapacitated from hospital relief and treated as a
vagrant.

4. Others said that there would not be objects enough in the
country to answer the purposes of a public hospital. But they
do not consider the great numbers that apply for relief in the
winter, suffering from dropsical, rheumatic, paralytic, and
scorbutic diseases, and slow and intermitting fever; and they do
not consider the cases requiring surgical operation, which have
to be removed by waggon to London (a three or four days
journey), after they have been fortunate enough to procure
letters of recommendation and a promise of admission.

These answers give a further insight into the motives behind the
establishment of voluntary hospitals, the advantages of which were
widely publicized. In an essay on the benefits of such institutions by
the Governors of the Winchester County Hospital the inadequate
existing medical provision for the poor was emphasized. Attention
was also drawn to the monetary advantages of giving a donation to a
hospital rather than to an individual and great stress was laid on the
religious benefits to be gained from hospitals. This was probably a
result of the still pervading attitude that sickness was an affliction
from God to be borne in the best possible spirit; it was perhaps also
accounted for by the presence of high-ranking clergymen on the
Board of Trustees. The two principal reasons given for supporting
these charitable institutions were both philanthropic and ulterior in
motive. Of sixteen reasons, the fifth stated that:[25]

It is incapable of being so far abused or misapplied, as to make Any One repent of their Bounty; which will appear to Those Who consider that, tho' the greatest part of the income should really be perverted, there would still be more good done by it, than by a larger Sum in any other manner. For a thousand persons will be relieved here at a less expence, than would be required for an hundred in the ordinary way of giving Alms.

The eighth stated that:

It provides for the relief and comfort of Multitudes who are unable to be at the expence of Advice or Physick, but are not distinguished by the name of THE POOR, because They do not come under the care of a Parish or Workhouse; and yet are the principal objects of this Charity, and most of all entitled to the regards of the Public; since They are in present want; and are of the diligent and industrious, that is, of the useful and valuable part of all Society.

These and similar arguments were used throughout the country in the formation of voluntary hospitals. An appeal for an infirmary at Liverpool included the following statement:[26]

Any one that fully Views the deplorable State of the helpless Poor, labouring under all the Variety of Diseases and Accidents, Calamities to which the legal Provision is confessedly inadequate, will immediately see, and admire The Usefulness of this excellent Design. In this calm Retreat they are provided with the neatest Accommodations, have the best Medicines administer'd under the best Direction, are served with the most convenient Diet, and meet with every Thing that human Aid can furnish for their Support and Recovery. These Helps, also, tho' not obtainable in any other method at any Price, are, as Experience evinces, here procured at the most moderate Expense: For any Contributions thus collected, and providently manag'd, become equivalent to much greater Sums dispensed in a private Manner; and the larger the Collection is, in a still greater Proportion are the Effects seen.

In London there was another early hospital which undoubtedly gave momentum to the voluntary hospital movement, though, strictly, it was not a voluntary hospital itself. Thomas Guy, a bookseller and a Governor of St Thomas's Hospital from 1705, announced in 1721 that he was going to erect and endow a hospital for incurables, thus 'establishing an asylum for that stage of languor and disease to which the charity of others had not reached, providing a retreat for hopeless insanity, and rivalling the endowment of kings'.[27] Although founded for incurables, the institution (opened after his death in 1725) was allowed to accept other patients and this role became predominant very quickly. The hospital followed the lines of the chartered hospitals because of Guy's enormous benefaction which enabled it to operate without the need of voluntary subscriptions. Two other people, John Radcliffe, who died in 1714, and John Addenbrooke, who died in 1719, left part of their fortunes to help establish hospitals in Oxford and Cambridge respectively, but their hopes were not realized until some years after their deaths.

In Scotland two attempts had to be made to get the first voluntary hospital established in Edinburgh. Alexander Monro, then a teacher of anatomy at the Surgeons' Hall, inspired by his father, wrote a pamphlet in 1721 on the necessity of there being a hospital in Edinburgh:[28]

> As Men and Christians we have the strongest Inducements, and even obligations to this sort of Charity, as it is warmly recommended and injoyned in the Gospel as one of the greatest Christian Duties: That Humanity and Compassion naturally prompt us to relieve our Fellow Creatures when in such deplorable Circumstances as many are reduced to, Naked, Starving, and in the outmost Distress from Pain and Trouble of Body and Anguish of Soul; That as the Relief of these is a Duty, so it is no less Advantage to a Nation, for as many as are recovered in an Infirmary are so many working Hands gained to the Country: That students in Physic and Surgery might hereby have rather a better and easier Opportunity of Experience than they have hitherto had by studying abroad, where such Hospitals are, at a great charge to themselves, and a yearly loss to the Nation: And as a Proof of the whole, they appealed to the good effects of the Infirmaries in all other Civilized Nations.

Though the sentiments expressed in the proposal were very similar to Bellers's original essay and to the thoughts of the authorities at the Westminster Infirmary and Winchester County Hospital, the effort by the Monros failed to receive the support needed, and it was not until 1725 that a second, successful, appeal was launched. The dispensary started by the College of Physicians had been a great success, but they found the premises used cramped and insanitary and so issued an appeal for a proper infirmary. The sum of £2,000 was raised and on 6 August 1727 'An Infirmary or Hospital for the Sick was lately open'd at Edinburgh, being the First Hospital of that kind that ever was in Scotland'.[29]

From these small beginnings the voluntary hospital movement[30] continued to spread through the country in the principal centres of population during the eighteenth and the first half of the nineteenth centuries.[31]

3   Philanthropy or social enhancement

The foundation of voluntary hospitals depended largely on the enthusiasm of the local community. This enthusiasm was often engendered by the local clergy who, having a duty to visit the sick and the opportunity to travel, became well acquainted with the condition of the poor. Alured Clarke, who was connected with the establishment of the County Hospital at Winchester, was also responsible for the foundation of the Devon and Exeter Infirmary.[1] His sermons on behalf of hospitals were printed and distributed throughout the country, for example, the third edition of the sermon he preached at the opening of the Winchester Infirmary was printed in Norwich in 1769 where a similar institution was proposed (actually founded in 1771).

At Northampton, Dr Philip Doddridge, a Nonconformist, and Dr James Stonhouse, a young physician, formally proposed a scheme in July 1743. A sermon on behalf of the proposed institution was given by Doddridge some weeks later and the hospital was opened in March 1744.[2] Dr Richard Grey, prebend of St Pauls, preached a sermon on its opening, reminding the congregation of the inadequacy of parish relief and the minimal cost of running such a charity. He added that 'The Government and Direction of it is in the Hands of Men of Character and Fortune; who have no Interest to serve by it, nor compensation for the Trouble they so generously give themselves, but the Satisfaction of Promoting a Publick Good'.[3] Doddridge had a great influence on Stonhouse, who was eventually ordained. Stonhouse preached on behalf of the Salisbury Infirmary in 1771 and is said to have compiled its statutes in 1766, though the movement at Salisbury had been initiated by a bequest of Lord Feversham.

St George's Hospital probably had the most aristocratic sponsorship: the first president was the Bishop of Winchester who was followed by the Prince of Wales and then by other members of the royal family. On the initial subscription list there was a number of bishops and a collection of nobility and other notables, including Lord Chesterfield, Lord Burlington, Lord Bathurst, Sir Robert Walpole and Garrick. At Bristol the group involved in the

17

foundation of the infirmary included a number of medical men, wealthy Quakers and others, including a John Elbridge, a Collector of Customs, who left the infirmary £5,000 on his death.

Members of the medical profession, as well as the clergy and nobility were involved in the establishment of hospitals. The prime mover of the London Hospital was John Harrison, its first surgeon. At a time when only 100 guineas had been guaranteed and the viability of the project was in doubt, Harrison announced to a meeting of interested people that the Duke of Richmond had become a subscriber, thus setting the seal on the worth of the institution. The Birmingham General Hospital was principally the work of Dr John Ash. 'The new ferment in their profession aroused medical men to the importance of institutions for treating the sick and studying disease, and they were quick to recognize and, in some degree, to guide the humanitarian sensibilities of their age.'[4]

Once the initial impetus had been given to a hospital, it had to achieve financial stability. The principal source of finance came from the subscriptions promised by the interested members of the community. This was the basis of the voluntary hospital system as the state aid advocated by Bellers had not been forthcoming. There were a number of inducements to attract a potential subscriber. According to the size of the subscription, usually ranging from one guinea a year upwards, he could nominate a certain number of patients, both in and out, to the hospital during the year.[5] A subscriber had the right to control the administration by the use of his vote at a general meeting and by having the power to elect the managing board for a yearly term. He also had the privilege of serving as a House Visitor to inspect the administration and day-to-day running of the hospital.[6]

There were other sources of income to supplement the revenue from subscriptions, which was liable to fluctuate from year to year. Donations, benefactions and bequests were very important to the hospitals, often saving them from closure.[7] Those who gave 25 guineas or more at one time received the benefits of subscribers for life. Large benefactions over £1,000 were usually invested in property or stocks to provide additional income and in times of difficulty could be sold to boost income.

A popular form of fund-raising was a music festival or an evening of entertainment. The hospitals in Yorkshire held shares in the Assembly Rooms in York and used the revenue to add to their income. The Birmingham General Hospital 'was mainly supported by Triennial Musical Festivals, at which such works as Mendelssohn's

"Elijah" conducted by the composer himself, and numerous other compositions of high merit written expressly for the Birmingham music meetings, were performed'.[8] Another pleasurable source of revenue was the annual dinner on behalf of the hospital. At the London Hospital the anniversary sermon was followed by a dinner in a hall of a city company or a tavern. The first dinner raised £36 14s. 0d., while in 1856 the sum had reached the record figure of £26,000. Sermons preached on behalf of the charity were another source of revenue: 'It is with Pleasure we Notice the continued Support the Charity receives from the ready Exertions of the Clergy of the different Denominations in this Town and Parish, and the consequent Collections.'[9] Though in the nineteenth century, this practice was not so common: 'As congregational Collections afford those who are not Governors an opportunity of contributing their offerings to this work of Christian love, it is much to be lamented that Sermons, which once greatly aided the pecuniary resources of the Charity, are now seldom preached on its behalf.'[10]

An innovation in fund-raising came in the middle of the nineteenth century with the advent of the Hospital Saturday Fund and, later, the Hospital Sunday Fund. From the 1850s collections had been made among workmen to support their local hospitals; the principal aim of the Hospital Saturday Fund was 'to collect small weekly subscriptions from the classes who cannot give considerable sums at one time'.[11] Each group involved in the Hospital Saturday Fund scheme had the rights of individual subscribers, while the Hospital Sunday Fund was a centrally-organized body whose aim was to stimulate church collections for hospitals and to distribute the funds received.

In spite of these other fund-raising measures, the subscriber was still the mainstay of the voluntary hospital movement. Why did individuals subscribe to these institutions? Were they persuaded solely by the benefits hospitals gave to a previously neglected section of the population? There were two non-philanthropic motives which could have influenced the potential subscriber, one spiritual, the other temporal. The sermons preached on behalf of the hospitals reflect on the Christian righteousness of giving to these institutions:[12]

To substitute hope for despair, to alleviate the poignancy of unexpected distress – to soothe affliction – and to administer comfort on the bed of despondency and sickness – are actions which every generous mind must feel a pleasure in performing:

It is yours to distribute these blessings around you, and yours to enjoy the satisfactory result.

Thus the subscriber would be helping his cause on the Day of Judgment. This is shown also in the suggested prayer for patients at Guy's Hospital – 'Bless all the worthy Governors of this hospital; excite in our hearts a grateful sense of their charitable care for our welfare, and grant that they may plentifully reap the reward of their labour and love, both in this life, and that which is to come.'[13] The involvement with religion pervaded all aspects of the hospitals' work:[14]

> To be at once Sick, or Lame, and Poor, is an afflicting Circum-
> stance indeed – and it certainly ought to dispose me, according
> to the Abilities God has given me, cheerfully to do my Part, as a
> Physician, a Christian, and a Subscriber towards your Cure,
> Instruction and Support. – But as Charity to the Soul is
> unquestionably the noblest of all Charities, I would especially
> attend to THAT; heartily wishing so to join the happy Purposes
> of a REFORMATORY with those of an INFIRMARY, as not only to
> restore your bodily Health, but effectually to promote your
> spiritual Welfare, and eternal Salvation.

The conscience of many individuals may have been salved by becoming subscribers for 'many a gambler and society miscreant found solace in channelling part of his ill-gotten gains to the cause of the sick poor'.[15]

Temporal inducements were connected with prestige and social status, a subscriber of whatever amount could have his name associated with the nobility and men of position in the community. It was possible for a small subscriber to become a vice-president or to attend all the social gatherings of the hospital, thus raising his social position. At Salisbury Infirmary, for example, a thanksgiving service was held in the cathedral to mark the successful completion of the first year:[16]

> Great preparations were made for the occasion, and those
> taking part met at the Council House in the City at half past
> ten. The Governors and subscribers to the Hospital were
> present, together with the Mayor and Corporation. It was
> decided that all should walk in an orderly procession from the
> Council House to the Cathedral being met there by the Dean
> attended by Officers of the Church. . . . On arriving at the West

Door of the Cathedral, the Lord Bishop of Salisbury joined those present for the service at eleven o'clock taken by the Dean. Afterwards, the procession . . . returned to the Infirmary where the Auditor's report was read. The gathering then witnessed laying the foundation stone of the permanent building by the Duke of Queensberry, the ceremony being concluded by a prayer composed and read by the Rev. D. Dodwell standing under the Cathedral standard. The day's events were brought to an end by a dinner at the Assembly Rooms in the City at two o'clock. All those who had taken part in the procession, including 149 Governors, were invited. The day's events, the procession, later known as the Infirmary Walk, and the Cathedral Service were repeated each year.

Anyone with social pretensions could not fail to enjoy such a gathering.

A subscriber to one of the English hospitals had a very strong inducement to give money as the right of admission into the hospital was virtually in his gift. There were seemingly strict rules which governed the right of admission:[17]

Ordered That a Subscriber of One Pound per Annum shall be allowed to have one Out-Patient on the Hospital-Book at a Time, and no more; and that a Subscriber of two Pounds per Annum shall be allowed one Out, or one In Patient at a Time, and no more; and a Subscriber of three Pounds per Annum shall be allowed one Out and one In Patient at a Time. That a Benefactor, who at one Time has given to the Infirmary, the sum of Twenty Pounds, shall be equal to an Annual Subscriber of two Pounds; and so in Proportion for greater or less Sums.

The size of the initial subscription and the rights it carried varied from hospital to hospital and over time, but the subscriber had a bargain by contributing to a hospital, as the cost of treatment, on average, exceeded the size of the subscription. The only method of gaining entrance to an English voluntary hospital was by the recommendation of a subscriber unless the sick poor person had suffered an accident or was considered to be an urgent case for other medical reasons. In Scotland the situation differed in that, in addition to the subscribers, a group of managers also had rights to recommend patients for admission.[18]

A contemporary view of the charitable characteristics of the English nation was that 'the English . . . are . . . the most devoted to

C

sympathy and commiseration, most tenderly alive to the softest impressions of every affection, most given to those emotions which flow from disinterested pity and concern . . . their courage is national instinct, and their charity is national refinement'.[19] From today's standpoint this statement would probably be considered naïve, but criticisms of the subscribers' motives does not detract from the fact that for the first time medical provision was being made available to the sick poor.

4   Hospital staff

Physicians, surgeons and apothecaries

The professional staff appointed to the voluntary hospitals occupied honorary positions and received no salary. In the chartered hospitals a salary had always been paid to the staff, but the sum did not increase over the years to take account of the changing value of money or the increasing responsibilities. There were a number of compensations for holding an honorary appointment at a hospital, the principal one being prestige; many of the hospital staff built up profitable private practices based on their success in the hospital, distinguished doctors would take on such duties as their own personal contribution to the relief of the sick poor,[1] and there was also the opportunity of becoming the physician or surgeon to the members of the governing authority of the hospital. The physicians and surgeons usually met once a week to admit patients and to see their patients in the wards:[2]

> each Physician and Surgeon attend alternately by their Weeks, to take in Patients on the Days of Admission . . . their Business on the Days of Admission be, to report the Condition of the Patients recommended to the Governors who attend, but they shall not take in, except there be no Governors present.

The physicians and surgeons for their trouble received similar benefits to the subscribers. It would appear that the duties of the staff could hardly be described as exacting: in 1820 at St Bartholomew's the physician had to attend the hospital only twice a week:[3]

> Each went his complete rounds once a week only. On another day he saw a crowd of out-patients, new cases, which were admitted only on that occasion . . . and any old cases in emergency. In his absence, his patients, as well as those of his two brother officers, were nominally under the care of the very worthy and very little apothecary of the hospital . . . The patients were really under the care of such of the physicians' pupils as considered themselves qualified.

23

The experience of the General Infirmary at Leeds was not uncommon, where some of the staff did attend frequently, but the minute books all too often recorded 'Neither Physician nor Surgeon here today'. In 1777 Dr Bird, one of the physicians, was asked to explain his frequent non-attendance. In a letter to the Board, Dr Bird begged 'leave to inform them that it is his Intention to attend the Infirmary as frequently as his private Employments will admit of'. This explanation was accepted by the Board and he was asked 'to accept the Office of Physician to this Charity for the Year ensuing'.[4]

What qualifications were needed for such demanding duties? Educational opportunities for potential physicians were very sparse, both in the number of training facilities and the quality of that training. The universities of Oxford and Cambridge originally held a complete and rigid monopoly in the education of physicians. The training was not of a very high standard, and the best physicians studied at the continental universities, particularly Leiden, although Paris, Montpellier, Bologna, Padua and Rome also taught medicine. The period required for medical training was excessively long and not really suited to practical medicine: a doctorate in medicine at Oxford originally needed fourteen years' attendance at the university, passing through the various stages from Bachelor of Arts to the ultimate achievement of Doctor of Medicine. This could be described as a liberal education as a candidate had to defend questions on logic, grammar, rhetoric, moral philosophy, natural philosophy, geometry, metaphysics, optics, physics and history. The medical education was principally a study of the classical authors, including the works of Galen. Lectures in physic and anatomy, botany and chemistry were perfunctory and there was no practical instruction at the English universities. Most medical students, however, went to one of the foreign universities where they obtained their M.D., and on their return they were able to 'incorporate' the degree at Oxford or Cambridge.

The Scottish universities, at Edinburgh, Aberdeen, Glasgow and St Andrews, all had medical faculties, but it was only the faculty at Edinburgh which had any real significance. The faculty of medicine was established in 1726 and by the end of the eighteenth century there was systematic and clinical teaching in medicine, surgery and midwifery, and practical instruction in natural history, botany and pharmaceutical chemistry. There was also an influential school of anatomy and surgery outside the university. The examination for the M.D. degree as enacted in 1767 was far more rigorous than the equivalent degree at Oxford or Cambridge, covering anatomy, surgery, chemistry, botany, materia medica and pharmacy, the theory and practice of physic, and clinical instruction given in the Infirmary. A candidate had also to present a medical thesis, written and defended in Latin. It is necessary, however, to add the qualification that the Edinburgh degree could be granted 'in absentia' if a candidate presented letters of recommendation from two physicians and offered a suitable thesis with the prescribed fees.

Oliver Goldsmith, writing in 1759, made certain comparisons between the standards of Edinburgh and Oxford:[5]

> Skill in the professions is acquired more by practice than by study, two or three years may be sufficient for learning the rudiments. . . . The man who has studied a profession for three years, and practiced it for nine more, will certainly know more of his business than he who has only studied it for twelve. . . .
>
> Four years spent in the arts (as they are called in colleges), is perhaps laying too laborious a foundation. Entering a profession without previous acquisitions of this kind, is building too bold a superstructure. . . .
>
> Edinburgh only disposes the student to receive learning; Oxford often makes him actually learned.
>
> In a word, were I poor, I should send my son to Leyden or Edinburgh. . . . Were I rich, I would send him to one of our own universities. By an education received to the first, he has the best likelihood of living; by that received in the latter, he has the best chance of becoming great.

At the General Infirmary at Leeds, for instance, of the first five physicians four were graduates of Edinburgh and one of Leiden, though graduates of Scottish universities were not entitled to practise legally in England until the Medical Act of 1858.

The standard of medical education rose dramatically with the advent of the voluntary hospital movement. In the university towns use was made of the new hospital facilities; the Governors of the Radcliffe Infirmary, Oxford, resolved in 1770 that 'the Physicians and Surgeons of the Infirmary be respectively desired to prepare a plan, to be laid before the Governors at their next meeting, for the admission of students in Physic and Surgery to attend the Infirmary'.[6] The professional staff in the hospitals were allowed to take on apprentices in their respective skills; this was a great perquisite for the staff as, for example, at the Bristol Infirmary in 1737 the apprentices had to pay a premium of 20 guineas for their seven-year apprenticeship. The fee was progressively raised until it reached 150 guineas by 1813. In 1758 each surgeon was permitted to bring two of his private apprentices into the hospital, and, in addition, the Infirmary had a surgical pupil who was apprenticed to all the surgeons. 'The profession quickly recognized the use of hospitals for teaching and also the value of those intangible assets which went with a hospital appointment. The pupils paid fees and, when duly fledged, recommended to their chiefs patients who could afford a consultation.'[7]

Towards the end of the eighteenth century the importance of hospitals for teaching medical students was increasingly being recognized and a number of institutions put their teaching on a regular basis. Manchester Infirmary, in November 1793, issued an invitation to potential students:[8]

> The Physicians of the Manchester Infirmary, Dispensary,
> Lunatic Hospital and Asylum, desirous of communicating the
> opportunities of instruction afforded by the extensive plan of
> these institutions, propose to admit pupils on such terms as to
> place the means of acquiring the most valuable information
> within the reach of persons in moderate circumstances. At the
> same time the nature of the practice offers peculiar advantages
> to those students who are enabled to seek for improvement in
> the knowledge and treatment of diseases wherever it can be
> found.

One of the regulations read that 'No persons shall be admissible as medical pupils but those who are or have been apprentices to Surgeons or Apothecaries or who shall have otherwise acquired the elements of medical knowledge by some preparatory course of regular education'.[9]

To fill the gaps in training, particularly in surgery, private medical schools had been established in London.[10] Perhaps the most famous school was that of William Hunter in Great Windmill Street, founded in 1768, where a thorough course in anatomy and physiology was given. The schools were often dependent on one person and on his death the institution would either lose its former reputation or close completely. In the nineteenth century provincial medical schools arose around the hospitals in Birmingham, Bristol, Hull, Leeds, Liverpool, Manchester, Newcastle, Sheffield, and York, as the training given by the universities was still weak.

The distinctions between the three grades of hospital staff, the physicians, surgeons and apothecaries, were very rigid and of considerable antiquity. The Royal College of Physicians was incorporated by Henry VIII in 1518 to control the practice of medicine within a seven-mile radius of London. Its primary purpose was to license recognized physicians who would thereby be distinguished from those who were unqualified; and it immediately established a monopoly. It was a professional guild of the elect, a college in the sense of 'providing a learned atmosphere for persons with similar interests and a joint determination to enhance the standing of the profession'.[11] The colleges of Edinburgh and Ireland were also closely connected with their respective universities. Surgery was not considered to be a respectable profession, and it only gained acknowledgment with the development of its own institutions in the late eighteenth century.[12] Each body developed independently of the others, having no formal links. Apothecaries, the only salaried members of the professional staff of hospitals, broke away from their fellow Mystery of Grocers in 1617 and established their right to treat the sick during the plague of 1665 when many of the physicians moved with their wealthy patients to the country. The apothecaries gradually extended their function from merely keeping chemists' shops to compounding prescriptions and the prescribing for and the treating of patients in their own homes. By the Medical Act of 1858 apothecaries were listed with physicians and surgeons in one register of medical practitioners.

This division between the various members of the profession was perpetuated by the hospitals in their ruling:[13]

> That no Physician or Surgeon belonging to the Infirmary,
> presume to order or intermeddle with the Patients, who are not
> under his own Care, except desired by the Person to whom they
> belong: And that no Physician, Surgeon or Apothecary, not
> duly elected by the Trustees to attend the Infirmary, be admitted,
> on any Pretence, to examine the Patients.

And again:[14]

> The practice of the physician, as it is universally understood, as
> well as by the College as the public, is to be properly confined
> to the prescribing of medicines to be compounded by the
> apothecaries; and in so far superintending the proceedings of
> the surgeon as to aid his operations by prescribing what was

necessary for the general health of the patient and for the purpose of counteracting any internal disease.

This contemporary view of physicians emphasizes their supreme position in the hierarchical structure of the medical profession. The peculiar practice of surgeons:[15]

> consists in the use of surgical instruments in all cases, and in the care of all outward diseases whether by external applications or internal medicines. Several diseases which may sometimes be regarded as internal complaints have been recognized as within the scope of their practice – syphilis, letting of blood, drawing of teeth . . . of customable diseases, as of women's breasts being sore . . . stone, strangury . . . all wounds, ulcers . . . fractures, dislocations and tumours etc.

The apothecaries' duties in hospital were more arduous than those of the physicians or surgeons as the apothecary was the only full-time resident member of staff. The basic duty of apothecaries 'consists in preparing with exactness and dispensing such medicines as may be directed for the sick by any physician lawfully licensed to practise physic'.[16] In a hospital the apothecary had far more to do; he was in charge of the daily bleedings, scarifyings, cuppings and blisterings; he supervised the baths and, where there was one, the new electrical machine; he looked after the surgical instruments; and he often acted as secretary, pharmacist and dispenser. The apothecary was very much the underprivileged member of the medical profession; the hospitals took advantage of the situation, and his duties were rigorously laid down in the rules:[17]

> That he dispense no Medicines, without the Direction of the Physicians or Surgeons, except in Cases of Necessity, when they cannot be consulted. . . . That the Physicians and Surgeons be at Liberty to inspect the Drugs and Medicines made use of by the Apothecary, and to see that he does his Duty; and that they enter their Observations in a Book to be provided for that Purpose. . . . That the Apothecary be never absent, when the Physicians and Surgeons are to attend, and that he always leave Notice with the Matron, or at the Place of his Abode, where he may be found, and in case of Sickness, or other necessary Avocation, that he depute another Apothecary, who shall be approved by the Physicians, to officiate in his Place.

The apothecary was the keystone of hospital practice by virtue of his constant attendance. As hospitals increased in size the duties of the apothecary became enormous, and in 1813 at the General Infirmary at Leeds the apothecary complained to the Board 'that the Business of the Hospital exceeds his Ability'.[18] As a result, in future years, assistants were employed to help the apothecary, though throughout the period under review the apothecary shouldered the main burden of responsibility in the hospital.

Matrons and nurses

The matron and nurses of a hospital were employed not as medical attendants but as servants. The matron as we know her today is quite unlike the matron of a hospital in the eighteenth and the first half of the nineteenth centuries. The most accurate description of the duties of a matron would be to take them as being those of a house-keeper. She had not, and was not expected to have, any experience of nursing. Her duties were designated in the rules of the hospitals:[19]

That the Matron take Care of the Household Goods and Furniture, according to the Inventory, and be ready to give an Account thereof, when required. . . . That she visit the Wards and Offices every Day, and take Care that the Chambers, Beds, Cloths, Linen and all Things within the Infirmary be kept clean. . . . That she keep a daily Account of the Provisions and other Necessaries, ready to lay before the Weekly Board, that she attend to the due Distribution of them, and never suffer any to be carried out of the House. . . . That she keep a Diet-Book, by which the Number of Patients on each Diet may be known. . . . That she cause the Names of the Patients in each Ward to be called over every Morning and Evening, and enter in the House-Visitors Book the Names of those who are absent, and that she suffer no In-Patient to go farther than the Inner-Court, without leave. . . . That she take Care of the Keys of the Doors, and see that they be always locked at Nine in the Evening from Michaelmas to Lady-Day, and at Ten in the Evening from Lady-Day to Michaelmas. . . . That she see that the Nurses, Servants, and Patients, observe the Rules of the House, and do their Duty; and in Case of Misbehaviour, or Neglect, acquaint the Weekly Board, or House Visitors thereof: That she never be absent from the House at the same Time with the Apothecary; and that she be free from the care of a Family.

What sort of woman would accept these duties? The main

requirements of a matron appear to have been respectability, middle age and, of prime importance, no family responsibilities. The first matron of the Salisbury Infirmary had previously been the assistant matron at the Winchester County Hospital; her letter of application read:[20]

> Hoping you will accept my services in admitting me to undertake the employment of a matron in your General Infirmary for which honour you may assure yourselves you shall never have cause to repent, for there is nothing from the kitchen to the garrett but I understand both to give directions and to do, as I have been so long in this Hospital, tho' I shall not make our Matron my example in all things. But I would not doubt of saving the House many pounds a year.

She was an exception in that she had had previous experience in a hospital, for most matrons were more than likely to have been 'in service' before their employment in a hospital. Over the years the duties and requirements of a hospital matron barely changed. In 1852 the General Infirmary at Leeds advertised for a new matron:[21]

> Candidates for this office are required to be free from the care of a family, of middle age, active, and of good address, qualified to keep an account of the disbursements and other matters in the house department; it is necessary that she be staid, sober, and discreet, mild, and humane of disposition, at the same time possessed of firmness to rule the household; it is also desirable that she be experienced in the management of a family and the duties of a sick room.

This was the first time that experience in nursing was mentioned, though, in a subsequent advertisement in 1862, this requirement had been dropped. It was not until the influence of Florence Nightingale pervaded the hospital walls in the late 1860s that superintendents of nurses were appointed who took over the management of the nursing staff, while the matron retained the duties of housekeeper.

Nursing in the eighteenth century was an unskilled profession, demanding little intelligence or aptitude, though it is interesting to note that in 1730 a list had been drawn up of the ideal requirements of a nurse:[22]

> Tho' it is impossible to meet with a Nurse every way so qualified for the Business, as to have no Faults or Failings, yet

the more she commeth up to the following Particulars, the more
she is to be liked. It is therefore desirable that she be:
1. Of middle age, fit and able to go through the necessary
Fatigue of her Undertaking.
2. Healthy, especially free from Vapours, and Cough.
3. A good watcher, that can hold sitting up the whole course of
the Sickness.
4. Quick of hearing, and always ready for the first call.
5. Quiet and still, so as to talk low, and but little, and tread softly.
6. Of good sight, to observe the Pocks, their Colour, Manner,
and Growth, and all alterations that may happen.[23]
7. Handy to do every Thing the best way, without Blundering
and Noise.
8. Nimble and Quick a going, coming and doing every Thing.
9. Cleanly, to make all she dresseth acceptable.
10. Well-tempered, to humour and please the Sick as much as
she can.
11. Cheerful and pleasant, to make the best of every Thing,
without being at any time Cross, Melancholy or Timorous.
12. Constantly careful, and diligent by Night and by Day.
13. Sober and Temperate not given to Gluttony, Drinking, or
Smoking.
14. Observant to follow the Physician's orders duly; and not to
be so conceited of her own skill, as to give her own Medicine.
15. To have no children, or others to come much after her.

This rather long list of desirable attributes tended to be acknowledged
in the rules of hospitals, though no mention was made of training or
knowledge of sickness. Nurses were thought of as servants and even
came below the cook in terms of salary. It was under the heading of
'Servants' that the regulations on nurses were given:[24]

That the Nurses clean their respective Wards by Seven in the
Morning, from the first of March to the First of October, and
by eight in the Morning, from the first of October to the first of
March; and that they serve up Breakfast, within an Hour after
the Wards are cleaned. . . . That the Nurses and Servants obey
the Matron as their Mistress, and that they behave with
Tenderness to the Patients, and Civility and Respect to
Strangers. . . . That all Persons concerned as Servants in the
House, be free from the Burden of Children, and the Care of a
Family.

The view usually held about nurses in this period is that they were the worst sort of women and that every vice was rampant among them. Even Florence Nightingale commented that nursing was generally done by those 'who were too old, too weak, too drunken, too dirty, too stolid, or too bad to do anything else'.[25] However, it should be remembered that it was only the bad cases which were mentioned in the minute books and reports, the good hard-working nurses were rarely praised for their diligence. Certainly, nurses were not the most scrupulous of women on occasions. It was known for nurses to extort money from patients for various services, though this was specifically against the rules, and at Guy's Hospital it was claimed that 'the salaries of the nurses and other servants were fixed at a considerably higher rate than in any other hospital, the better to prevent their extorting money from the patients'.[26] Nevertheless the nurses must have acquired some medical skill just by being in the wards, and it was said that the sisters of St Bartholomew's in 1830 had 'an admirable sagacity and a sort of rough practical knowledge which was nearly as good as any acquired skill'. Through experience nurses must have learnt how to dress wounds, how to relieve pain by suitable applications and by changes in posture, and some would have learnt how to interpret patients' symptoms and thus gauge the seriousness of particular cases. An advertisement from Salisbury Infirmary in 1796, when there was a shortage of nurses, pointed out 'the advantages to young, strong, respectable women who would be taught how to look after sick people'.[27]

In *Martin Chuzzlewit* Dickens assures the reader that 'not the least among the instances of their [the hospital's] mismanagement that Mrs. Betsy Prig is a fair specimen of a Hospital Nurse'.[28] A defence of the nurse, though rather ingenuous, came from Lord Granville who stated that 'the nurses are very good now, perhaps they do drink a little, but so do the ladies' monthly nurses, and nothing could be better than them: poor people; it must be so tiresome sitting up all night'.[29]

Surely, the hospitals got as good a nurse as they were prepared to pay for and to offer decent working and living conditions. *The Times* of 1857 commented:[30]

Hospital nurses have been much abused – they have their
faults, but most of them are due to want of proper treatment.
Lectured by Committees, preached at by chaplains, scowled on

by treasurers and stewards, scolded by matrons, sworn at by surgeons, bullied by dressers, grumbled at and abused by patients, insulted if old and ill-favoured, talked flippantly to if middle-aged and good-humoured, tempted and seduced if young and well-looking, they are what any woman might be under these circumstances.

The pressure on nursing staff became increasingly acute in the nineteenth century with the growth in the numbers and the size of the voluntary hospitals and the change in the scope of treatment. Initially, moves were made to eliminate the cleaning duties performed by the nurses. In 1856 the Nursing Committee of Salisbury Infirmary recommended 'that in future the wards be cleaned and scoured by persons engaged for that purpose and your nurses kept in every particular distinct and separate from the servants of the establishment'.[31] The next step was to provide trained nurses, and the same recommendation continued: 'It is hoped that the establishment of Institutions for the training and education of nurses will afford the Infirmary the means of introducing by degrees an improved system into the hospital.'[32] A year earlier than the recommendation from the Salisbury Infirmary, Liverpool Royal Infirmary had considered the role of nurses in the hospital:[33]

Upon the punctuality of the nurses, in observing the directions of the medical officers, depends mainly the success or otherwise, of the treatment; whilst, by proper surveillance, they may be the means of preventing much waste in the wards, and, by their general deportment, exercise a most beneficial influence on the patients themselves. Your Committee are of opinion that the experience necessary to constitute a good nurse can only be obtained by a course of previous systematic training and discipline for the duty; and it has been from a deep conviction of the advantages to be derived therefrom that they have acceded to an application from the managers of the recently formed ' "Nurses" Institution', to allow a limited number of probationers access to the house during the day, in order to acquire that knowledge in the treatment of disease, in its varied forms, and method in the management of the sick, for which no place so well as the interior of a large and well regulated hospital affords such ample opportunity.

At this time:[34]

powerful advocates of reform appeared among the humane public, the clergy, and to some extent the medical profession, and, as was natural, the foundation of an English Order of nursing became the objective. . . . In circular letters and public addresses the religious foundations of the past were quoted for the virtues of their leaders, and if no familiarity was exhibited with the weaknesses revealed by the records, there was a fervent wish to reproduce the accomplishments. Fruitful results followed the exertions of small groups of zealous women, fixed with the common impulse of love for their fellows, and well supported by persons in high positions or distinguished in the worlds of philanthropy or literature.

Elizabeth Fry, of prison-reform fame, founded the English Protestant Sisters of Charity in 1840, though the 'Protestant' part of the title was soon dropped and the institute in time gained access to hospital wards. The Salisbury Infirmary placed its nurses under a Nursing Superintendent from this institution in 1857. Perhaps the most important of the other communities was that of St John's House which was established in 1847 under the aegis of Sir William Bowman, the ophthalmologist and surgeon to King's College Hospital. The pupil-nurses attended the hospital and received instruction from the medical staff, including the physiologist, Robert Bentley Todd. In 1856 the Order took over the nursing at the hospital:[35]

> so as to introduce a higher class of nurses and a better system of nursing into the wards of the hospital, and to carry out more fully than hitherto one main object of the St. John's House institution – that of training and providing nurses for the sick in hospitals, as well as for private families and the poor.

The All Saints' Community founded in 1856, though it had nothing to do with the original movement, was responsible for the nursing at University College Hospital for over twenty years from 1859.

It was not until 1860 that the Nightingale Fund Training School was founded in connection with St Thomas's Hospital. Florence Nightingale endowed the institution with the money given to her by the nation as a token of gratitude for her services in the Crimea. The principles on which the training was based were sobriety, honesty and truthfulness, but the former religious virtues were not insisted upon. A nurse had to be clean, quiet and punctual; she had to look after the patient in a personal manner; and as an assistant to the medical staff the nurse's duties were defined so that she could be of help at the bedside. The administrative aspects of hospital life were to be learnt by day-to-day routines for cleaning, heating, etc., and the domestic side was to be mastered by lessons in cooking and laundering.[36] The function of the Nightingale School, as it happened, was more to train matrons than to train nurses.[37] Her pioneer spirit, encouraged by her widespread pupils, allowed the hospitals to establish their own training schemes,[38] but there was a distinction between the lady-pupils, who paid for their training, and the probationers, who were paid. It was from the lady-pupils that the sisters in charge of the nurses usually came:[39]

> No longer was nursing regarded as a superior form of domestic service which did not always attract respectable members of the 'servant class'. It had become a vocation: it had become a proper occupation for daughters of the middle and upper classes. . . . There is no reason to doubt that the medical care of the patients was greatly improved. The patients also enjoyed greater physical comfort. On the other hand they must have felt a certain loss of homeliness in the wards for which the kindly intent of the new nurses did not compensate. . . . The homely, dirty, foul-mouthed nurses must sometimes have been missed.

5   Admissions policy

The limited hospital facilities available at the beginning of the eighteenth century were to be expanded considerably because of voluntary subscription during the century. From the opening of the Westminster Infirmary in 1720 to 1760 five general hospitals, three lying-in institutions and two special hospitals were founded in London. This was the limit of hospital development in London until after the turn of the nineteenth century when three general hospitals and eleven special hospitals were established to 1840. In the provinces there were no general hospitals in existence before 1735, by 1760 there were 16, by 1800 38 and by 1840 no less than 114. In 1861 there were 23 voluntary teaching hospitals and 130 voluntary general hospitals in England and Wales.[1] The peak period of construction in the eighteenth century appears to have been between 1735 and 1775, when 21 hospitals were established. The movement in the provinces followed that in London; only 9 of the provincial general hospitals had been founded by 1745, the date of the establishment of the last general hospital to be founded in London in the eighteenth century. By the end of the eighteenth century there was a hospital serving all the principal centres of population with the notable exceptions of the West of England and Wales.[2]

The number of beds available in the voluntary general hospitals in 1800 in England was approximately 4,000,[3] of which about one-half were in London. By 1836 'the number of beds which the London and Provincial Infirmaries of England, altogether contain, is about 6,850',[4] while for 1861 the number had risen in England and Wales to 11,848, of which 3,662 were in London.[5] The number of beds available may not seem very great by today's standards for the size of the population. England and Wales had a population of about 9 million in 1800, 14 million in the mid-1830s, and 20 million in 1861.[6] This figure of 1861 meant that the number of beds in voluntary general hospitals per thousand of the population was 0·59.[7] But is this low figure for the whole population really significant? The facilities offered by hospitals were only available to a small part of the population, i.e. 'the deserving poor', those who not only had no other access to medical provision but were also members of the working population. It was these people who were in real need, the section of the population who were most likely to be susceptible to disease and illness. In addition, each bed was available for more than one patient per year as the average length of stay varied between thirty and forty days.

Contemporary descriptions of conditions in towns are by any standards quite horrifying; the urbanized population had expanded rapidly without an adequate increase in the number of dwellings, resulting in a high density of population and worsening hygienic conditions, all of which was conducive to an unhealthy environment. The area in which the Westminster Hospital had been established was peculiarly prone to flooding and it became notorious for fevers, malaria, typhoid and 'infectious diarrhoea'. The congested houses were a perfect setting for tuberculosis not only of the lungs but also of the skin and of the bones. When St George's Hospital broke away from the Westminster and took Lanesborough House at Hyde Park Corner, one of the reasons given was that it was:[8]

far enough for the patients to have the benefit of a country air;
which in the general opinion of the physicians would be more
effectual than physick in the cure of many distempers,
especially such as mostly effect the poor, who live in close and
confined spaces within these great cities.

The pioneers in medical advance noticed the connection between poverty, urban squalor and disease: 'Great cities are like painted sepulchres; their public avenues, and stately edifices seem to preclude the very possibility of distress and poverty; but if we pass beyond this superficial veil, the scene will be reversed.'[9] These few lines indicate the conditions prevailing in the cities and the points are reiterated by one of the physicians to the Manchester Infirmary who wrote that 'the mean lodging-houses . . . are the principal nurseries of febrile contagion'.[10] These sentiments were echoed more forcibly and in more detailed terms in the famous sanitary reports of the nineteenth century, where the life of the poor was described in all its harrowing detail.

Though it is necessary to emphasize the dreadful urban conditions of the time, it should be remembered that, according to the position of the hospital, country patients were equally important. Naturally, the London hospitals were immediately concerned with their

D

neighbouring poor, but the provincial hospitals always had a large intake of patients from the surrounding countryside. The General Infirmary at Hull reported that:[11]

> the population of Hull is, like that of the kingdom in general, rapidly on the increase. The reputation of the INFIRMARY stands deservedly high, and patients, especially surgical ones, have sometimes come to it from a considerable distance on that account. There being no General Hospital nearer than Leeds, it is the recipient of the sick from all the surrounding country, the access from which to Hull has been facilitated almost beyond calculation, by the introduction of steam-boats, through which the whole tide of population on the Humber, and its tributary streams, pours in its diseased poor.

Hull, being a sea-port, also had 'a class of Patients, to which this Institution has long extended its beneficial aid, that of Foreign Sailors'.[12] Liverpool, a city which was burdened with poor housing, surprisingly found that in 1750 two-thirds of the in-patients at the Infirmary came from the country and from Ireland.[13] The General Infirmary at Leeds reported in 1785 that a number of prospective patients had to be turned away because of its inability to accommodate them; the large number of applications was due to 'the Increase of our Manufactories and our numerous Applications from distant Places'.[14] Of the hospitals in Scotland, the Edinburgh Royal Infirmary stated that 'the Charity is not confined to the City of Edinburgh, or to any particular Counties or Burghs'.[15] In the first year of its existence patients were admitted not only from Edinburgh, but also from such scattered places as Caithness and the Isle of Mull.[16] The Dumfries and Galloway Infirmary found that patients from the county of Galloway usually comprised only about one-third of the total admitted.[17]

The distinction should be drawn, when looking at the places from which patients were accepted, between general and county hospitals. County hospitals usually restricted their intake to patients from the surrounding area, while general hospitals had no specific rules regarding place of residence and were prepared to accept patients from outside the county boundary.[18]

A prospective patient, in England, needed the recommendation of a subscriber before he could be admitted to a hospital. The subscriber could be an individual, a township or a parish, and the sick person had to find one of these who was willing to certify that he was 'a proper object of the Charity'. This was the only way of gaining admittance to a hospital unless the prospective patient had been involved in an accident or had symptoms which needed immediate relief. At the two royal institutions of St Bartholomew's and St Thomas's, and at Guy's, each individual case was considered separately and at the London Hospital, in addition to the usual method of admission, a sick person could 'petition' to be treated on the payment of a penny. In Scotland the procedure for admission was somewhat different from English practice. The regulations of the Aberdeen Royal Infirmary were typical of the other institutions in Scotland: 'The persons entitled to recommend patients to the Infirmary are, the Managers of the Hospital, the Clergy of the several parishes and congregations who contribute annually for the support of the House, and those who individually subscribe for the same purpose'.[19] Thus, although individual subscribers had the rights of admission, as their English counterparts, there was an additional section of the local population who had the right of recommending patients. The Managers, who administered the running of the Infirmary, were partially elected to their position, while others automatically became Managers on their appointment to several of the important positions in the city.

Once a sick person had surmounted the first hurdle of finding a subscriber prepared to recommend him, the potential patient also had to find a deposit to defray the cost of his burial if he were to die in the hospital – 'That No In-Patient be admitted without bringing a Security from some Substantial Person to defray the expenses of Burial or Removal'.[20] This ruling was not universal, though it was more frequently practised than not. The Westminster and the London Hospital did not require deposits and the Leicester Infirmary dropped its demand for 12*s.* caution-money in 1773, though a prospective patient then had to bring a certificate signed by the Overseers of the parish to which he belonged that they would remove him from the Infirmary on notice being given and would pay the funeral expenses in the case of death.[21] Many hospitals varied their policies over the years with regard to caution-money, for example, at Addenbrooke's Hospital, Cambridge, it was agreed in 1766 'that no Security shall be taken for the Burial of Patients',[22] but by 1778 the ruling for patients coming from a distance was that they should acquire 'some Person to engage to pay the Funeral Expences of any such Patient who shall happen to die'.[23] The ruling of the Infirmary at Bristol was similar: 'that Persons recommended, whose place of residence is ten miles distant (Sailors and Casualties excepted) shal Deposit 12/- with the apothecary to defray the Expence of the Funeral in case they Die, or for their Removal in case they are Discharged'.[24] Differential rates were applied from 1797 according to the distance the patient lived from this Infirmary, reaching a peak of 40s. for a patient who came from over thirty miles distant – 'The surplus remaining after defraying the expences of removal, or, in the case of Death, the funeral, to be returned to the Friends or Overseers, whoever shall have made the deposit.'[25]

There were still further conditions attached to entry of a hospital. Patients were supposed to be admitted in a clean condition and having a clean set of clothes: 'It is particularly desired, that all subscribers recommending patients, do take care that they are sent clean, and free from vermin; and that they bring with them, at the time of admission, three shirts or shifts, and other necessaries for keeping them clean.'[26] Charges were sometimes made for the laundering of bed-linen, etc.; the General Infirmary at Hull ordered that 'Every in-patient must deposit with the Secretary ten shillings, which will be repaid when the patient is dismissed; deducting the expenses of washing'.[27] The ruling by 1850 had become even more comprehensive: 'Patients shall bring with them Changes of Linen, a Plate, Basin, Knife, Fork, Spoon, Soap, and a Towel, and provide for their Washing.'[28] At Bristol Infirmary the authorities were visibly more compassionate as one of the early minutes records 'that no Patients be taken in till their Cloaths are well cleansed, and where any of them are so poor that they can't pay for it, that the visitors of the Week do order the matron to pay for doing it'.[29] Sheffield General Infirmary followed this example in 1800: 'Resolved – That a discretionary power be vested in the Weekly Board, to order the washing of the Linen, at the expence of the Charity, of such Patients only, during their continuance in the House, as are entirely destitute of the means of procuring it themselves.'[30]

The last set of restrictions concerned the type of person who could be admitted into a hospital. The classification of the 'deserving poor' or 'worthy objects of charity' usually excluded servants, apprentices, and the like as well as the most obvious category of 'pauper'. It has been said that a subscriber often gave money to a hospital so that his 'sick servants need never be on his hands',[31] but there were usually special rules about servants as they were considered to be able to receive treatment through the good offices of their masters. The General Hospital in Birmingham put its position most diplomatically in a statement of 1779:[32]

> no domestic servants shall merely on that account be excluded the benefit of the Hospital, but it shall be left to the determination of the Committee, how far the servant is, or is not, a proper object. The Committee are always to consider it is contrary to any institution of this nature to relieve those who are able to pay for their cure; and it is reasonable to hope that all masters (whether subscribers or not) who are in affluent circumstances and have hitherto been accustomed to pay for their servants, will not desire them to be relieved at the public expence, to the detriment of more necessitous objects.

As experience was gained in the administration of a hospital practice varied over time and from hospital to hospital. The original rule of the Winchester County Hospital, for example, was 'that no Domestick Servant of a Governor or Principal Subscriber, shall be relieved at the Hospital, except in such particular cases as shall make a Person incapable of continuing in Service'.[33] However, in the late 1820s a statement was issued to the effect that:[34]

> it having been the custom for a length of time to make the moderate charge of One Shilling a Day for the Board of In-patients, who are servants of such individuals as may be considered from their situation in life, able to bear the expence, and the finances of the Hospital, being relieved by this practice; the Committee wish it to be generally understood that it is left entirely to the discretion of the employers of such servants either to reject the charge, if the payment should be deemed inconvenient; or to remit the amount to the Secretary; and thereby become Benefactors to the Institution.

The General Infirmary at Leeds amended its rules soon after its opening, when it was resolved 'that the Servants and Apprentices of such Persons as are in Poor Circumstances and would avail themselves be thought proper to be Admitted Patients into this Infirmary shall for the future at the Discretion of the Weekly Board be admitted Patients notwithstanding their being Servants or Apprentices'.[35] It was found, however, that there were a number of difficulties attached to this ruling and a subsequent minute noted that:[36]

It is the Opinion of the Board, That the 39th Rule should stand as it does, to prevent the admission of Gentlemen's Menial Servants who are not truly discharged from their Service, at the Time they are of Opinion that when Servants have voluntarily relinquished their Engagements with their masters and being in very distressed circumstances cannot procure Relief from their Masters, that such Servants are real Objects of Charity and cannot consistently with the design of this Charity be rejected as Patients.

The General Infirmary in Hull specifically excluded apprentices by a ruling of 1850: 'No Apprentices, whose Master or Mistress is in circumstances to pay for their cure, shall be admitted as Patients.'[37] In Scotland the Edinburgh Royal Infirmary extended the benefits to the inhabitants of being able to admit their servants. They:[38]

are liable to sickness and accidents – they may be seized with contagious diseases, when it would be unsafe to accommodate them in their own homes. The Royal Infirmary affords the means of seeing every faithful servant, under the pressure of pain or disease properly cared for, and his case treated by medical practitioners of ability and experience.

Though parishes often made subscriptions to hospitals to enable their poor to receive treatment, paupers who were dependent on the parish for their livelihood were not permitted to be recommended: 'It is requested that no subscriber will recommend any patient from a Parish Workhouse, as no person under that description will be admitted.'[39]

There were two further categories of patients where special rulings applied, supernumerary patients and soldiers. Supernumerary patients were peculiar to the Edinburgh Royal Infirmary, and were taken in over and above the number of patients which the institution could afford to have at any one time. It was ordered that 'Supernumerary patients, that is, those exceeding the establishment of ordinary patients, shall pay sixpence per day till vacancies offer'.[40] Soldiers were only accepted normally if the cost of keeping them in the hospital was paid. The ruling at the General Infirmary at Leeds was typical: 'That Soldiers resident in Leeds, who are destitute of Medical Help, may be admitted Patients of this Charity upon due Recommendation; and that such of them as are deemed proper for In-Patients, do pay Four-Pence a Day so long as they remain in the

House'.[41] The Manchester Infirmary laid down a specific rule about
the admission of soldiers, which other hospitals followed: 'That no
soldier be admitted as In-Patient, until his Officer has engaged to
pay his Subsistence Money to the Treasurer of the Infirmary during
such Time as he shall continue there, except Soldiers on Furloe,
when there is no Officer at hand to engage for them'.[42]

Thus, entry into hospital was bounded with many restrictions,
which narrowed the section of the population for which the medical
facilities were available. What were the occupations of those who
did manage to conquer these barriers? At the Salop Infirmary for
the year 1845–6 there was a wide range of occupations, from
agricultural labourers to prostitutes, from writing clerks to quarry-
men and stone-cutters.[43] This was representative of a small provincial infirmary located in a primarily agricultural area, though the
extraction of natural resources was represented by miners and
colliers, etc. In the large manufacturing towns the bulk of the
patients, both in- and out-patients, were people employed in the
factories, though factory workers were often admitted for accident
rather than for disease contracted through bad working conditions.
Every hospital found that the process of industrialization put
increasing pressure on their resources. In Sheffield the General
Infirmary found that in the middle of the nineteenth century
'An increased and increasing population, the proximity of railways, the continued introduction of complicated machinery,
rendering accidents more frequent, tend continually to augment
the necessity for a larger amount of accommodation in the
Infirmary.'[44] A physician advancing the cause of hospitals in
manufacturing areas at the beginning of the nineteenth century
commented that:[45]

In advocating the cause of wards for the sick poor in
manufacturing districts, it has been much the practice to advert
to the numerous factories, not merely as a source of
accidents, but as conferring a degree of unhealthiness on those
whom they employ. There was a time indeed, when those springs
of wealth, especially the cotton factories, were nurseries of
disease, and thousands of victims were immolated at the shine
of avarice; but both in the woollen and cotton factories, a
most happy change has taken place, and such is the attention
to ventilation and cleanliness, as well as to the general comforts
of their inmates, that it is doubtful if in so large a mass of

individuals working at their own houses, you would find so small a proportion of sickness.

This point is further underlined by a commentator on the Manchester Infirmary, writing in the 1830s: 'The sub-acute character of the diseases of the manufacturers is strongly demonstrated by the fact, that of 1,046 patients admitted into the Manchester hospital in the year 1832, and whose occupations were registered, only 208 belonged to the factory classes.'[46] These comments would imply that it was the environment rather than the nature of the work which contributed to disease. The remark of the Sheffield General Infirmary concerning the accidents from the construction of railways was repeated time and time again, wherever a railway was being constructed. At the Northampton General Hospital, for example, it was reported in 1835 that 'the number of beds had to be increased to 112 because of the number of serious accidents during the construction of the London to Birmingham railway, particularly at Blisworth and Kilsby'.[47] The hospitals in the sea-ports of Britain tended to admit large numbers of cases of accidents received by dockers and seamen, while the London Hospital was founded specifically to relieve 'Poor Manufacturers, Sailors in Merchant's Service, and their Wives and Children, with Medicine and advice in case of Sickness or Accident'.[48]

Thus, from the little information available, it would appear that the voluntary hospitals served the section of the population in greatest need, the 'deserving' labouring poor.

6 On the books

That no Woman big with child, no Child under Six Years of Age, (except in extraordinary Cases, as Fractures or where Cutting for the Stone, or any other Operation is required) no Person disordered in their Senses, suspected to have the Small-Pox, Venereal Disease, Itch, or other Infectious Distemper; no Persons apprehended to be in a dying condition or incurable, be admitted as In-Patients, or if inadvertently admitted be suffered to continue.[1]

This formidable list of exclusions is in addition to the special qualifications for admission already discussed, and is representative of the admissions policy of voluntary hospitals in the eighteenth and nineteenth centuries. Dr Doddridge, preaching on behalf of the Northampton General Hospital in 1745, having studied the reports from the hospitals at Winchester, Bath, Exeter, York, Bristol and the London and Westminster hospitals commented that he found 'palsies, dropsies, consumptions, fevers, leprosies, rheumatisms, cholicks, stone, as well as multitudes of ulcers, fractures, dislocations, and the like, on the list of those calamities from which these poor creatures have been relieved'.[2] This list of cases appears to include some of the excluded diseases and therefore a question must be asked as to its representative nature. The rules of the different voluntary hospitals followed basically the same pattern as those quoted, being modified occasionally in the light of experience. It appears that the rules were generally designed to exclude the chronic sick and the cases which were likely to prove troublesome in one way or another. Hospitals were loath to admit cases which were likely to prove infectious;[3] the exclusion of pregnant women and children is again associated with the fear of the spread of disease. Puerperal fever was likely to arise where pregnant women were giving birth to their children, and children are naturally more susceptible to disease as they have not developed immunity of any kind.

Some hospitals did accept pregnant women under special circumstances. When the Middlesex Hospital was established, a lying-in ward was proposed and opened in 1747, but it was closed in 1807 for reasons of economy. At the London Hospital the treatment of maternity cases was authorized from its opening:[4]

> Mr. Cole, the Apothecary to this Infirmary, also followed the Practice of Midwifery, having proposed to attend every Wednesday in the Afternoons from 3 to 5 for the Relief of Women with Child and the Distempers incident thereto, Agreed that he do attend accordingly, and give them the necessary Advice and Relief.

A proposal was made in 1790 by three surgeons and one physician of the Manchester Infirmary to establish a scheme to deliver poor pregnant women in their homes, but it was not adopted and the four people involved resigned and founded what eventually became St Mary's Hospital. However, the Infirmary did adopt a plan a few year later to offer 'assistance to POOR MARRIED WOMEN In difficult labour'.[5] In Scotland the Edinburgh Royal Infirmary opened a lying-in ward in 1755, where a limited number of maternity cases were treated free of charge, but a small fee was charged for super-numerary cases. The ward was closed in August 1793 when a separate building was provided for maternity patients. The Dumfries and Galloway Infirmary passed a resolution in 1789 'that under certain regulations, poor married women, in the last month of their pregnancy, who may wish to be taken care of, and delivered at the Infirmary, shall when properly recommended, be received into one of the upper wards of the House, and there duly attended for the time that may be necessary'.[6] These few hospitals which made arrangements for pregnant women were the exception rather than the rule, though lying-in hospitals were established in London during the eighteenth century.

Exceptions were made about some of the other exclusions at various times. Chronic cases were not normally admitted, but this was knowingly done on occasions. An early statement from Liverpool Infirmary was that 'many inveterate and desperate cases presented themselves at the first Opening, and have, while there was room, been admitted without Exception – This, by God's Assistance will not be the Case hereafter'.[7] The Dumfries and Galloway Royal Infirmary came under pressure during the 1820s:[8]

> By the rules of this, as well as of similar Institutions, the admission of Patients labouring under disease which afford no

reasonable hope of cure, is strictly prohibited; but since the pressure on the labouring classes became so severe, the number of cases of hopeless consumption, under the most miserable circumstances of destitution, has become so great and urgent, that the Committee could not, on the score of humanity, deny to many of them such a refuge from their sufferings, as the Infirmary afforded.

Sheffield General Infirmary reported on similar problems a few years earlier when it found that 'such is the measure of distress in this neighbourhood, that the Wards of this Hospital have recently been unusually filled, and in various instances occupied by persons who have known better days'.[9] This class of patient was normally excluded and the authorities at the Manchester Infirmary emphasized the point in an early annual report to their subscribers: 'CON-SUMPTIVE and Asthmatick Persons in general being more capable of receiving Relief without Doors, It is desir'd that Subscribers for the future will not recommend them for In-Patients'.[10]

Infectious disease was always a problem with the hospital authorities. Again, a hospital had to make its policy clear in a statement to its subscribers: 'Persons suspected to have the itch cannot be admitted In-Patients'.[11] This same hospital, the Birmingham General, experienced trouble with chronic patients of a particular type; it reported in 1783 that:[12]

the Beds have been constantly filled with Patients, many of whose cases were of such a Sort as to prove tedious in their Cure. . . . Patients with sore Legs of long standing will always prove a heavy Burden upon a Charity of this Nature, and particularly so, from the various Arts that some will practice to protract their Cure, in Spite of the utmost Vigilance of the Surgeons.

Patients with habitual external ulcers were a further category which presented hospital authorities with problems. The usual practice was to exclude them as their cure was rather prolonged and the patients, therefore, took up scarce beds for far too long, though some institutions did change their rules subsequently to assist these cases. One such was the Salisbury General Infirmary which, in 1828:[13]

Resolved, that it should be left discretionary in the Committee, on recommendation of the Surgeons, to admit habitual Ulcers, of long standing, at present excluded by the sixth rule for the admission of Patients, for a period not exceeding three weeks, for the purpose of putting such Patients in a way of managing themselves; but that such Patients shall be discharged by the weekly Committee at the expiration of such three weeks.

A class of patients which caused the hospitals more problems than any other were those who suffered from venereal disease. It was considered the worst form of punishment for the sins of the flesh and the transgressions of Christian morality deservedly resulted in the sufferers' afflictions. The practice concerning these cases varied and in general it was considered improper to admit them. A committee was formed at the Westminster Hospital in 1736 to investigate the practice prevailing in the other London hospitals and to find the best method 'to prevent the entertaining of any patients who have contracted their distemper by drinking gin or other spirituous liquors and to desire them to co-operate with this Society in discountenancing that most pernicious practice'.[14] A subsequent report in 1739 concluded that 'Inquiry of the large Hospitals found that venereal patients were either not admitted at all or only upon an extraordinary contribution to their support. Any in-patient therefore being found with venereal disease is to be discharged immediately without awaiting cure.'[15] It was not until 1834 that a ward was set aside for syphilitic women in this hospital. The position at the General Infirmary at Leeds was considered in 1775:[16]

The Trustees having been often obliged to exclude from the Benefit of this Charity, Persons who appeared to be innocent Sufferers by the Venereal Disease, when their Cases required Admission into the House; as all Persons afflicted with this Disease, by what Means soever, were incapable of Admission, according to the 44th Rule; it was judged proper to make such an Alteration in that Rule, as might suit the benevolent Designs of this Institution; without exposing the Patients to the injurious Society of debauched Persons, whom that Rule was intended to exclude. At a General Quarterly Board held June 28th 1775, it was therefore ordered, 'That married Persons of good Character, and Children of such Patients, afflicted with the Venereal Disease, be admitted In-Patients of this Charity, on due Recommendation'.

In London a Lock Hospital had been established in 1746 for the treatment of patients suffering from venereal diseases, and there were wards allocated for the treatment of such patients at the Winchester, Manchester and Leicester infirmaries.[17]

The regulations on the admittance or not of infectious diseases and fevers caused the hospitals a great deal of trouble. These cases were generally excluded from hospitals, as once they were admitted there was the continual problem of checking the spread of the disease. However, there were exceptions and hospitals were often dilatory in dealing with the problem effectively; thus at the Birmingham General Hospital, one of the largest provincial institutions, it was not until 1830 that 'separate Wards for the reception of infectious or offensive cases' were completed.[18] The separate House of Recovery, built in Manchester, for the treatment of fever patients was said to have 'been the means of diminishing the sum of disease, and consequently of misery and of death'.[19] At the Newcastle Infirmary fever cases were admitted until 1774, from which date they were excluded from the building.[20] In 1790 the Salisbury General Infirmary decided to accept the victims of an outbreak of smallpox, but within a month it was ordered that 'patients having small-pox in the Infirmary be forthwith removed to some proper place and that all the expences of removal and care be paid by the Infirmary'.[21] By 1803 the Infirmary had become less generous, as one of the physicians stated that 'a patient has been seized with small-pox and has been removed to the Pest House, ordered that all expence attending her removal be paid by the Infirmary, and the cost demanded from the parish of Knoyle'.[22] Practice regarding the admission of fever cases varied considerably in the provincial hospitals, while in London the two royal institutions and Guy's Hospital accepted them, as did all the hospitals in Scotland.[23]

The differences in admission practices and the attitudes towards various diseases between the English and the Scottish hospitals is very clearly shown in the contrasting statements of John Aikin, the well-known physician in Manchester, and of an anonymous writer on behalf of the Edinburgh Royal Infirmary made in the 1770s.[24] Taking the comments of the writer at the Edinburgh Royal Infirmary first of all, the contrast becomes more striking with the statements of an English physician:[25]

Some diseases have been held improper for hospitals. Patients labouring under pulmonary consumptions, if the disease be

advanced to the second or last stage, will suffer from the air of
the hospital, however well ventilated. But, in the beginning of
the disease, while its nature is perhaps still equivocal, patients
of this kind may be admitted. Scrophulous cases, when of the
more inveterate kind, not admitting of a radical cure, are
improper for hospitals. But, if a physician wishes to try how
far palliation will go, he will find frequent opportunities.
Epilepsies, though hard of cure, ought to be taken under trial,
since they have been often found to proceed from worms alone.
Palsies and dropsies, when the patients are not beyond the
vigour of life, and more especially when the diseases originate
rather from an accidental than a constitutional cause, merit
admission. But when these diseases proceed from an advanced
age, and debilitated habit, they cannot be expected to admit of
a cure. After all, a physician will hardly choose to do so great
violence to humanity, as to reject a patient in very necessitous
circumstances, though he may be sure that patient is to die
under his care.

Seven years previously John Aikin had written about the same
subject, but with conflicting conclusions:[26]

No disease fills our hospitals, especially in some parts of the
kingdom, with so many surgical cases as the scrophula, and
none is in general more improper for admission. When this
virus has once infected the constitution it is continually showing
itself in numberless different appearances from the slightest
glandular tumour to the most inveterate pulmonary
consumption and white swelling of the joints.

He continued:

I have seen numbers of these miserable creatures, covered over
with ulcers, disabled in their limbs, and emaciated by
suppurations and pulmonary obstructions, applying for
admittance into a hospital, and received merely from the
forcible commiseration which their wretchedness excited.[27]

In this disease there seem to be no reasons for admitting into a
hospital sufficient to counterbalance those against it, except
where amputation is necessary on account of a joint swelling,
or in a few cases which render some other operation
advisable.[28]

Aikin was of the opinion that venereal cases should be treated, as the mercury used to 'salviate' these patients needed careful control, despite the fact that 'the operation of mercury, dispose the body to emit putrefactive effluvia which strongly tend to corrupt the surrounding air'.[29] As to cancer, he considered that:[30]

> There is so small a probability of curing it by any means hitherto discovered, and it is so loathsome an object to the senses, that unless the removal of the part affected by an operation be practicable and advisable, it can with no degree of propriety be received into a hospital.

Aikin had doubts about the efficacy of allowing scorbutic ulcers into hospitals and he concluded that 'It must be confessed that although the ulcers are brought to heal by the common hospital treatment, the cure generally only stands good while the confinement lasts'.[31] And he further argued that these cases were often sent away 'in a worse condition than they entered'.[32] On fevers, he argued that:

> EVERY fever, it is true, is liable to contract a malignancy from the bad air of a hospital, which also becomes communicable, but in many of them, such as the pleuritic, nephritic, rheumatic, and all of the like nature, this disposition is in so inferior a degree, that, unless the hospital be in so wretched a state as to deserve the name of a Pest-house rather than an Infirmary, there need be no scruple in admitting them.[33]

> ALL diseases affecting the lungs, are of that kind which can never receive benefit from even the sweetest and best contrived hospital.[34]

He saw hospitals as institutions for the acute sick and not the chronically ill which was the intention of the hospital rules; he 'would wish to enforce as much as possible the idea of a hospital being a place designed for the cure of the sick, and not an alms house for the support of the indigent and decrepid'.[35] It has been necessary to dwell at some length on the comments of the physician at Edinburgh and of Aikin to illustrate the difficulties facing hospitals in forming a policy for the admission of patients. The impression left by these opposing views is that Aikin was probably being too much of an idealist in a world of imperfect diagnosis, while the Edinburgh physician was being far more realistic about the types of cases seeking admission, and on a humanitarian rather than a medical basis thought that they should be admitted.

What cases did slip through the net of exclusion? The problems of diagnosis were great and most hospitals appear to have received unwittingly a number of pregnant women, epileptic and insane patients, patients suffering from venereal disease, lousy patients and some with smallpox. Pregnant women appear to have got past the admitting committees with some regularity. A rather sad case occurred at the Radcliffe Infirmary, Oxford, in 1777:[36]

> On Monday last died in our Infirmary, Martha Jewell, a young woman admitted about five weeks ago, under Pretence of a Dropsical Disorder: some hours before whose death, upon examining the Girl's Box under her bed, a female child was found wrapped up in a quilted petticoat, of which it appeared she had been privately delivered. On Wednesday an Inquisition was taken upon the body of the infant when the Jurors returned their Verdict of Wilful Murder against the deceased mother. From Circumstances upon Examination before the inquest; it appeared that she had been delivered eleven days before her death.

The Northampton General Hospital found that it had admitted a pregnant woman in 1771, and decided that she ought to be helped. It, therefore, 'Ordered that a proper lodging be taken to remove Ann Aldermante she being in child labour; also that necessary things are brought her for the child if born alive'.[37] The London Hospital was a little harsh with one of its female patients for 'Elizabeth Brazier, an in-patient, having been delivered of a female child in the House on Thursday morning last, Ordered, as its father could not be found, that the said child be sent to the Foundling Hospital immediately'.[38]

Smallpox, of the other excluded cases, presented recurring difficulties. Bristol Infirmary decided on its policy, a compassionate one, as one of its first acts and ordered:[39]

> That all In-Patients who are attacked in the Infirmary with the Small-Pox, be instantly removed from it, to proper Lodgings provided by the Matron, and that their respective Physicians, and in their Absence, some other Physician belonging to the House visit and take care of them, and that all such Patients be supported during such Illness at the Expense of the Society.

The London Hospital also did this if they discovered such a patient in the House, although the hospital did have a subscription to the Smallpox Hospital to avoid incidents of this kind.[40] A common practice was to send any smallpox cases which arose in the hospital to the local pest-house.

Epileptics were usually refused admission, not because no effective cure was available, but because of the effect on the other patients. Such was the case at the London Hospital where it was found, as in other hospitals:[41]

> that patients troubled with Fits are a cause of a great deal of Inconvenience in the House, not only by frightening in the same Distemper some who were never subject to it before, but also by frequently occasioning a Relapse to such as were almost cured, and as they can be treated as out-patients, Ordered to be treated as such.

Chronic cases kept on re-appearing, as at the Winchester County Hospital in the year 1804–5, which were admitted 'rather than they should die on their way back'.[42] The hospitals in Scotland did not escape this problem as Glasgow Royal Infirmary found that 'On some occasions no fewer than twelve beds have been occupied in such hopeless cases and thereby much unnecessary expence incurred'.[43]

If a patient proved a nuisance because of offensive smells and unpleasant symptoms, a hospital often ordered his removal and assistance was given as an out-patient. Thus, the Weekly Board of the Norfolk and Norwich Hospital in March 1778 ordered 'That Houghton, an in-patient, who is removed out of the house on account of an offensive mortification, be allowed such additional assistance as his case may require'.[44]

As the nineteenth century progressed the voluntary hospitals started to show a little more compassion towards the excluded cases by amending their rules to allow treatment as out-patients, though only if they had been admitted by mistake in the first place. The typical ruling read that 'if admitted inadvertently [the excluded cases] be permitted to continue, but that they be treated as Out-Patients, and assisted with advice, medicines &c'.[45]

John Clark, physician to the Newcastle Infirmary, made a number of statements about the application of the exclusion rule in provincial hospitals which shows up their inadequacy in the light of the contemporary demand for hospital services:[46]

E

This rule is taken from the London hospitals, where the patients recommended live in the vicinity; but such a rule must often be infringed, when applied to county infirmaries. When a patient is sent from a distance, and in so weak a state as to be unable to undergo a second journey, he must be admitted into the house, whatever be the nature or state of his complaint: Nay, even when a patient is able to return to his home, urged by the entreaty of the sufferer, and unwilling to offend a distant subscriber, who seldom makes use of his privilege of recommending, the receiving physician or surgeon cannot refuse admission. Hence the Infirmary is often crowded with patients, in the incurable state of many of these forbidden diseases; and any Governor, by taking a survey of the wards, will observe, that the house almost always contains a number of incurable diseases, and also a number of patients capable of receiving equal relief out of the Infirmary, although the latter are kept in express violation of the 16th rule.

He had some particularly relevant remarks to make about the admittance of fever cases which he found:[47]

often are received into infirmaries, masked under the form of rheumatism and catarrh: Nay, I will go further – Since I belonged to the Charity, I never rejected a patient because he laboured under evident symptoms of low fever: Other physicians, nay, I believe all of them, have done the same.

This would appear to have been a more realistic view of the situation in hospitals and would obviously reflect on the types of cases admitted.

The voluntary hospitals were under no legal obligation to publish lists of the cases treated, and thus usually confined their reports on the hospitals' progress to the total numbers only of those treated and discharged.[48] In the eighteenth century there were only a few instances of hospitals giving any public information on the diseases treated, but from approximately the middle of the nineteenth century the practice becomes almost universal with the introduction by William Farr, the Registrar-General, of a standard classification of diseases.

A comparison of the diagnoses for the eighteenth century with those of the second half of the nineteenth century illustrates the lack of diagnostical techniques available in the earlier century. Ausculta-

tion (sounding of the chest) and the use of the stethoscope or ther-
mometer were unknown to the physicians of the eighteenth century,
and even in the nineteenth century, the physician did not have the
benefit of X-rays, which did not come into general use until the first
quarter of the twentieth century to assist his diagnosis. Diagnoses,
by present-day standards, can only have been superficial, relying
on external symptoms and signs, and the complaints of the patient.
Thus, the amount of credence which can be placed, at least on the
early lists, is open to question.

The Worcester General Infirmary opened on 1 January 1746 and
in the following thirty-three months cures were claimed for
'Dropsies; Mortifications; Scrophulous, Scorbutick and Fistulous
ulcers; Empyema; Inflammation of the Eyes, with Albugo; Simple
and Compound Fractures; Saint Vitus's Dance; Rheumatisms,
some of twenty years' standing; internal Haemorrhages; Jaundice;
Tinen; Wound of the Selival Duet; Impetigo; Gunshot Wounds
through Part of the Liver; Pleuresy; Epilepsy'.[49]

During February 1734 St George's Hospital admitted cases of
consumption, intermitting fever, rheumatism, jaundice, herpes,
chlorosis, albugo, fractures, (external) ulcers, tumour of the breast,
caries of the leg, glandular tumour, ringworm, rupture, stone in
bladder, scorbutic eruptions, flux, contusion, gravel, worm fever,
pain in breasts, palsy, ophthalmis, fever, asthma, dropsy, colic and
spina ventosa. A further list from the same hospital for the period
from 1 January 1734 to 16 July 1735 shows similar complaints with
some additions. The cases include arthritis nodosa or knotty-joint
gout; leprous eruptions and leprosy; lues and lues venerea; foul
ulcers; scurvy manifesting itself in scorbutic rheumatism, eruptions
and ulcers; tumours; smallpox; St Anthony's Fire and St Vitus's
Dance. At one time a diagnosis is given as 'scrophula', at another
'the evil' or 'the king's evil', this disease usually displaying symptoms
of glandular swellings on the neck, eruptions on the face, or affections of the eye. As has been shown, the rules of the voluntary
hospitals apparently excluded infectious diseases, and yet in the list
cases of ringworm, scald head, whooping cough, chicken-pox,
scarlet fever, puerperal fever, itch, erysipelas and syphilis are to be
found. However, the list should be treated with care as it does not
discriminate between in-patients and out-patients.[50]

Cases admitted as in-patients during the first two months of
operation of the Westminster Hospital exhibited symptoms of ague,
obstructions, scurvy, asthma, dropsy, consumption, sciatica, palsy,

hysterical colic, scorbutic rheumatism, strain, carious bone in knee, leprosy, scrofula and evil in the head.[51] A report published by this hospital for the early 1720s contains such 'distempers' as 'schyrrhosity with Floodings', 'Old Cholick, tetterous Eruptions, Piles and Rheumatism' and 'Intermitting Fever, Bloody Flux and Looseness'.[52] These are some of the more graphic diagnoses, but the majority of cases appear to be of fever, consumption, scrophula, etc.; so much for the admissions ruling excluding precisely these sorts of cases.

The Bristol Infirmary, like many other hospitals, admitted a number of chronic cases despite a specific ruling to the contrary. This is illustrated by such diagnoses as 'Lowness of Spirits', 'Hypocondria', 'Pain of the Limbs', 'Pain of the Stomach', 'Mania', 'Scorbutus', 'Gravel' and 'Haemoptoe'.[53] A common form of diagnosis was recorded as 'Impostummation', which was used to represent any kind of abscess or inflammatory swelling. The admission and discharge registers for this hospital for the middle years of the eighteenth century show a prevalence of fevers, dropsy, pleurisies, pneumonia, rheumatism, painters' colic, scurvy and leprosy.[54]

When the cause of the Devon and Exeter Hospital was being advanced in 1741, evidence was taken from the experience of the Winchester County Hospital:[55]

> The poor themselves are next invited to observe that such long continued ailments as dropsies, colics, heart ailments, and the like, lasting for two and even three years, were capable not only of material alleviations but in some instances positive cure, when such rest, suitable food, and the best of medical skill were available as in such an hospital as was then being built.

The cases that were admitted to the Devon and Exeter Hospital between 1742 and 1777 were classified under the following headings: 'Leprosies'; 'Gutta Serena'; 'Cataracts'; 'Cancers'; 'Stone by Extraction'; 'Stone by Cutting'; 'Imposthumes'; 'Strumous and Scorbutic Disorders'; 'Dropsies, Colics and Asthmas'; 'Rheumatisms'; 'Paralytic Disorders'; 'Bruises, Fractures and Dislocations'; 'Wounds, Tumours and Ulcers'; and 'Epilepsies'.[56]

What were to become two of the largest voluntary hospitals in the North of England, the Manchester and Newcastle Infirmaries, published detailed reports on their early days. Manchester divided its patients into forty-two different categories, while Newcastle expanded its divisions to a total of forty-seven. The lists of cases from these two hospitals are very similar to those from the other hospitals. Some of the more unusual diagnoses were 'complication', 'surfeit' and 'uterine disorders' at the Manchester Infirmary, and 'falling sickness' and 'ruptures' at the Newcastle Infirmary.[57] Again, despite the exclusion rule, there was the presence of infectious and chronic cases. Thus, for example, at the Newcastle Infirmary there were in-patients suffering from 'consumption' and 'extreme weakness', and out-patients with 'scald head'.

The hospitals in Scotland fared no better. During the first year of operation of the Edinburgh Royal Infirmary, patients were received with disorders ranging from 'Consumption' to 'Pthisick and Tumor of the Belly after a Quartan Ague'. The same types of cases are seen, though the exclusion rule was not applied at this institution. Of interest is that four patients diagnosed as having cancerous growths on different parts of the body were admitted.[58] A comment on the admission to the Glasgow Royal Infirmary, which might well apply to all the voluntary hospitals, was that 'On the medical side of the House the diseases were limited very much to those of the lungs, heart and kidneys, and the fevers. . . . In these lists there is a good deal of overlapping and many of the diseases were simply the names of symptoms.'[59] The first patient received at the Royal Northern Infirmary, Inverness, on 3 July 1804 was 'Elspet Munro from the Parish of Urquhart, and was suffering from a scrofulous swelling upon the left knee'.[60]

Some unusual cases were admitted to the wards of the voluntary hospitals, including an extraordinary case at the Nottingham General Hospital. On 4 August 1783 Kitty Hudson was admitted as the ninth patient. She was a seamstress and over the years she had swallowed a great many pins and needles. Apparently large numbers of these objects and various bones were removed from her feet, legs and arms, and from other parts of her body. Both her breasts had to be removed, and yet she was dismissed as 'cured' on 12 July 1785.[61]

Naturally, the voluntary hospitals were not only treating in-patients, they also provided medical aid to out-patients. 'Dislocated shoulders, broken arms, bruises, scalds, crushed fingers, broken heads, injuries to eyes, or to hands, and great variety of accidents which do not necessarily interfere with the locomotion of the sufferer',[62] were given the assistance of treatment by the physicians and surgeons of the hospitals.

Once the voluntary hospitals had become established in their local communities, and as the number of patients increased, they tended to cease publishing detailed lists of the cases which were treated each year. As a result it is very difficult to gain an impression of the work of the voluntary hospitals in the first half of the nineteenth century. There were a few local studies of the activities of the regional hospitals and a hospital occasionally published a list of the diseases it had treated.[63] A government inquiry in 1834, requiring information for a commission into medical education, asked for details on the numbers of acute and chronic sick treated but not for any specific details of the diseases.

A survey made by the house surgeon at the Sheffield General Infirmary of the cases received from January 1798 to January 1820 concluded that the diseases prevailing among the labouring poor in the Sheffield area were 'Rheumatisms, Scrophula, Ulcus, Hernia, Gastrodynia, Amenorrhoea, Paralysis, Abscess, Cephalaea, Caries, Febris, Lumbago, Pleurodynia, and Vitia Cutis'.[64] In accident cases, 'Contusions, Fractures, Wounds, Burns, and Scalds' were the most frequent.[65] The author made some comments on the more interesting cases which are worthy of note. He found that of the asthenia cases many:

> were in a state of great feebleness, left by the sequelas of various acute diseases, and by difficult parturition, and old age. . . . A great many of these Patients suffered, apparently under Dyspepsia, brought on by irregular and poor living, and by a constant habit of smoking tobacco, and drinking spirituous liquors.

Under the category of 'Ophthalmia' was included every species of the disease 'and other defects of vision, which frequently accompany this disease. The greatest number of [the paralysis cases] were Hemiplegia.' 'Tussis' was described as a 'Constitutional or habitual Cough'. Of 'Vitia Cutis', the author found that many were 'of the various species of eruptive disorders'. Many of the 'Vulnus' (i.e. wounds), 'were very extensive contused, lacerated, and some gunshot'.[66]

This case-study demonstrates the most common diseases prevalent in a provincial infirmary in a manufacturing town. The diseases, despite the use of the Latin names, are virtually the same as those described for the eighteenth century, and are typical of the cases treated by the voluntary hospitals.

The one unusual characteristic of the cases received at the Sheffield General Infirmary was the presence of 'grinder's asthma', an occupational disease peculiar to the cutlery trade. A physician to the Infirmary made a study of the hazard in 1830 when he examined the cases he had treated between 1817 and that date. Of the 250 grinders he had treated, '154 were cases in which the respiratory organs were affected'.[67] As a comparison he examined 250 other patients (excluding grinders, boys under fourteen years of age and females) and found that 'only 56 had pulmonary complaints'.[68] He commented that the disease was usually fatal, while 'a large proportion of the pulmonary cases met within the second class consists of habitual asthmas, and chronic coughs; complaints which, though frequently incurable are seldom fatal'.[69]

If the Sheffield General Infirmary is compared with the Manchester Infirmary for a similar period, a bias of a different kind appears. Mill artisans were peculiarly prone to derangement of the digestive organs, and of the 5,833 patients under the care of a physician at the Manchester Infirmary between 1826 and 1830 the cases of dyspepsia, constipation and other affections dependent on derangement of the digestive organs, were more than one-third of the entire cases. Another peculiarity distinguishing the list was, that one-fifth of the number was made up of coughs, etc., while scrofula and consumption, in its varied forms, was exceedingly limited.[70]

From about the middle of the nineteenth century the hospitals appear to have exercised more control over their admissions, and it must be assumed that this was because of improvements in diagnosis. The diseases listed became more distinct and precise.[71] As diagnosis and knowledge about diseases improved, the classification of disease became more accurate, and the standard classification advocated by William Farr was taken up by most of the hospitals, though there was no compulsion for them to adopt the scheme, from the 1860s onwards.[72] The hospitals re-introduced the practice of publishing lists of the cases admitted, particularly after the inquiry into the voluntary hospital system in 1863.[73] Under the headings of the standard classifications the specific complaints were registered, thus giving a more accurate account of the experience of the hospitals. The diagnoses evidently became more accurate, no longer being mere descriptions, and the treatment increasingly specific. As these changes occurred the hospitals became more selective in their treatment of cases and adhered to the exclusion rules. The emphasis moved to the treatment of the acute sick and the diseases which were listed bear a much closer relation to the types of complaints which a hospital should treat. A medical practitioner today would probably be aware of the diagnoses given and would approve of the admission of such cases to the wards of a general hospital.

Thus, the voluntary hospital system from a faltering start in the eighteenth century, established itself in the nineteenth century as a series of institutions where, in the general hospitals, the acute sick could find effective treatment.[74]

7   Fever cases

The subject of the admission or non-admission of cases of fever is exceedingly complicated and the terminology is very complex.[1] The principal area of interest in this chapter is the practice of hospitals towards the admission of fever cases and not that towards the cases of fever which may have broken out within the walls of a hospital. The evidence would suggest that the practice with regard to fever cases varied from hospital to hospital and even from year to year.

The background to the provision of medical facilities for cases of fever is very limited. In London when there was an outbreak of the plague little was done in the way of segregation. Herbs were worn by the people to ward off the dreaded disease; and carts were sent round to collect the dead who were buried in specially dug pits. The wealthy tended to leave the city, thus taking the disease with them, but the poor had to remain and get what attention they could from the remaining physicians.[2] The two royal hospitals of St Bartholomew's and St Thomas's admitted the fever patients, but their accommodation was limited. The only other arrangements in London appear to have been the pest-houses in Finsbury and Westminster, which had been provided by the parishioners independently of any legal authority or obligation.

By the rules of the voluntary hospitals any form of infectious disease was excluded from entering the hospital, but despite the ruling a number of cases did get past the admitting physicians and surgeons, without their knowledge. Furthermore, there were a number of hospitals where, in spite of the rules, fever cases were admitted.

A physician, writing at the end of the eighteenth century on the achievement of hospitals at that time, made a number of observations about the treatment of fever patients:

In every Hospital, clean and well-aired wards should be
reserved for the separation of such patients as, from delirium,
contagious or putrid effluvia, or from any cause whatever,

61

might be hurtful to others; or such as themselves may require a better air for recovery. . . . Patients ill of fever should not, undoubtedly, lie near to those who are confined on account of fracture, wound, &c. It is, however, as clear, that patients with fever are of the last description that should be crowded together. The case, from its nature, demands more than ordinary attention to every circumstance relating to air. . . . The condition of patients of Hospitals in fever, so as far as relates to number in a ward, requires, generally, to be mended.[3]

The prohibition of contagious diseases, especially the fevers, cannot effectually secure any Hospital or Infirmary from the introduction of the contagion of fever; for it is known to lie inert in the body from a few days to a few weeks. A physician, indeed, may easily distinguish a contagious fever, when strictly formed; and so far the prohibition, in several instances, may have been useful in preventing its introduction into a ward: but, it must be observed, that before a physician can have an opportunity of ascertaining the real nature of any disease, the patient has remained for a considerable time in the waiting-room, crowded with other patients, some of whom may have received the contagion; and from this cause the infection has frequently been inadvertently received into the Hospital; and often has been spread, by the out-patients in waiting; widely into the country.[4]

This comment by the physician to the Newcastle Infirmary at the beginning of the nineteenth century shows the position of the hospitals at this time, the prevention of the admission of fevers into the wards was extremely difficult by the nature of the buildings themselves and the lack of diagnostic techniques. He continued:[5]

But the following is a much more frequent way in which fever is introduced into Hospitals without fever-wards. When fevers prevail in a town, or even subsist in a single infected house, poor persons, with latent contagion, apply for admission for, perhaps, a rheumatism, or a catarrh; no medical sagacity can detect the lurking poison. The patient is admitted – and the fever does not discover itself for some days, or weeks. If the Hospital be provided with a fever-ward, still, by removing the infected person on the first or second day of the fever, the rest of the patients in the ward may escape.

Clark was writing on behalf of separate fever wards at the Newcastle Infirmary and, therefore, had to present a formidable case, but his remarks have the ring of truth about them. Diagnosis was not exact and it would appear that it was possible for some forms of fever to be knowingly admitted by the physicians.[6] The Newcastle Infirmary had, in fact, forbidden the admission of cases of fever and contagious skin diseases by a special minute of the Governors in 1774.

In a letter to John Clark it was stated that in the London hospitals, 'particularly St Thomas's and Guy's fever cases are admitted – and so far from being kept in separate apartments, are distributed, in equal proportions, through the different wards; so little do they fear the propagation of contagion in a freely-circulating state of the atmosphere'.[7]

Other hospitals did inadvertently admit fever cases, such as the London Hospital and the Salisbury Infirmary.[8]

> The Liverpool and Manchester Infirmaries, although from their first institution the admission of fever was strictly prohibited, yet, in both of them, contagious fever was inadvertently received, and spread to so alarming a degree, that the patients were taken out of the wards, in order that they might receive purification.

Of the English provincial hospitals, it was only the Chester General Infirmary which received fever patients as a conscious policy, albeit into separate wards. The great reformer, John Howard, visited Chester and remarked that 'the two fever-wards were not in the least offensive: they were fitted up on the upper floor, on account of a contagious fever in Chester in 1784'.[9] The wards were opened at the instigation of John Haygarth, the physician to the Infirmary, who was a leading figure in the cause of treatment for fever cases. The rules he formulated for these two wards were extremely strict, and were based solely on the need for complete separation from the rest of the building and the other patients – 'No fever patients, nor their nurses, are suffered to go into other parts of the house. No other patient is allowed to visit the fever wards; nor any stranger, unless accompanied by the apothecary or his assistant.'[10]

The Manchester Infirmary had, in 1781, formulated the first positive policy of any of the voluntary hospitals towards cases of fever, but this did not involve the provision of separate accommodation for the patients. In that year it was decided to treat 'all such poor patients in their own houses that are afflicted with any contagious disorder such as the small-pox, measles, etc.'[11] In June 1790 a new building for out-patients was decided upon and the decision was made that the upper floor 'be so contrived as not to communicate with the Infirmary and to be set apart and kept ready in case any in-patient should be seized with a fever or other infectious disorder during his stay at the Infirmary'.[12] However, the decision on the fever wards was rescinded at the next meeting and it was not until 1796 that wards were opened as an annexe to the dispensary. John Ferriar, physician to the Infirmary, who campaigned for general improvements in public health, was instrumental in establishing a fever hospital in Manchester. As the result of an outbreak of fever in Ashton-under-Lyne in 1795:[13]

> A committee was formed for the relief of the sufferers, and a subscription was raised for supplying them with medicines, and wine. An attempt was also made, to provide a house for the reception of fever-patients, but from the general prejudices of the sick, it was impossible to procure their removal from their own houses.

A Board of Health was established after this outbreak of fever which gave impetus to the fever hospital movement, culminating in success in May 1796, when the so-called House of Recovery was opened:[14]

> Previous to the building of our Dispensary, when a patient happened to be seized with an infectious fever in the Infirmary, the disease was apt to spread to an alarming degree, so as to require a general dismission of the patients. But since a few rooms have been added to the Dispensary, for the purpose of secluding persons thus attacked, from the rest of the patients, though bad fevers have been accidentally introduced, yet by removing the patients, on the first attack, into the fever-ward, the disease has always been prevented from extending, without the necessity of dismissing a single patient.

The fever wards were an evident success:[15]

> To so great a degree have contagious fevers been reduced, since the establishment of the house of recovery, that the limits of the house are now extended to the whole of Manchester and its extensive suburbs, and to every point of the vicinage for two miles round, from whence a fever patient can be safely removed.

The success of the Manchester House of Recovery inspired other towns to follow suit, and the voluntary hospitals in general became more aware of their responsibilities towards cases of fever from the beginning of the nineteenth century. The opinion of the most eminent physicians of the day was that separate fever hospitals and fever wards should be established and that the notion of mixing fever cases with the other cases should be abandoned.[16]

The first separate fever hospital in London was opened in 1802 under its full name of the 'Institution for the Cure and Prevention of Contagious Fever in the Metropolis'. A contemporary commented: 'It is not a little remarkable that it should have been left for the opening of the nineteenth century, before an hospital for the cure and prevention of contagious fevers should have found an establishment in either the police or the liberality of this metropolis.'[17]

An outbreak of fever in Hull during the winter of 1803–4 encouraged the Trustees of the General Infirmary to open 'Two WARDS OF PREVENTION, to relieve those suffering from the effects of a contagious Typhus Fever, which has lately much prevailed, and to prevent its ravages in future'.[18] The Faculty of the General Infirmary also reported on the sanitary principles which should be observed in towns, concluding with the statement that 'By neglect of these and similar circumstances, diseases occasioned by the unwholesome state of the atmosphere, are increased in frequency and malignity'.[19]

It was as responses to outbreaks of epidemical fever that positive steps were taken to provide accommodation for and treatment of fever cases in many towns, such as Liverpool, where a fever hospital was opened in 1806 on the lines suggested by John Ferriar. 'The Parish appointed it for the reception of the poor when suffering from infectious fevers, and medical service was given by the physicians attached to the Infirmary.'[20]

Smallpox presented problems to the hospital authorities, both before and after the introduction of vaccination. Salisbury General Infirmary found that it had to provide accommodation for patients suffering from smallpox, despite the fact that a smallpox hospital had been established by the parish in 1763. The Trustees purchased the old County Gaol in 1822 to give the Infirmary room to expand, and in 1825 when smallpox and fever were prevalent in the city the Infirmary offered to vaccinate the poor free of charge and 'Part of the gaol lately used as a debtors' ward was let to the City for the purpose of receiving poor persons infected with the fever then prevailing'.[21]

The Radcliffe Infirmary, Oxford, had its own problems in 1818:[22]

> There has never been a detached building to which patients
> seized in the Infirmary with small-pox or other highly
> contagious disorder could be removed – any person seized with
> the small-pox in the Infirmary [were removed] to one of the
> pest houses in the House of Industry, the Infirmary bearing the
> expenses. . . . Twice within the last two years small-pox has
> appeared on persons admitted into the Infirmary, and the
> patients could not be accommodated in the House of Industry
> (as it was full) or in any other place without the Infirmary
> walls therefore they remained from necessity, and from
> necessity also in the body of the building. . . . The Governors
> of the Infirmary are anxious to prevent the recurrence of such
> an inconvenience by erecting two small wards, one for male, the
> other for female patients, at the north-west extremity of the
> back court of the Infirmary.

The building, called Hakewill, was opened in 1824. A separate fever
block was opened in the same year at Leicester General Infirmary,
and in 1828 a Special General Meeting of the Nottingham General
Hospital decided:[23]

> that additional Wards should be erected for the reception of
> patients afflicted with contagious and other diseases. These have
> been erected on a spot adjacent, but contiguous to the South
> West end of the present Hospital, and will be opened for the
> admission of patients on the 25th of June [1828].

The rules of admission to the fever block at the Nottingham General
Hospital were typical of the period and are particularly notable for
the lack of separation between the various febrile diseases.[24]

The cholera epidemic of 1831–2 gave hospital authorities a lot of
trouble and each coped differently with the situation. The principal
policy was one of exclusion. Thus, at the Salisbury General Infirmary
the Governors 'were of opinion, that in the present state of the
country it is not prudent to admit any vagrants into the Infirmary,
and that no cholera patients be received',[25] despite the appeal of the
local Board of Health for the Infirmary to turn the fever wards over
to cholera patients. In the later cholera outbreak of 1849 it was
ordered in July of that year 'that all persons labouring under
premonitory symptoms of cholera should be admitted as out-
patients without a recommendation paper'.[26] During this period

only three patients in the Infirmary were struck with the cholera and they were removed to special lodgings for treatment. In Oxford the Radcliffe Infirmary supplied drugs at cost price to the cholera hospital at Pepper Hill during the first outbreak, while in the outbreak of 1854–5 cases were admitted to the special Hakewill building:[27]

> The outbreaks of Cholera in 1832 and 1849 [in Hull], again demanded special vigilance on the part of the authorities at the Infirmary, not however in the nature of preparations to receive Cholera cases into the House [as the rules of the house forbade the admission of contagious disease], but to guard against, or be prepared for any case arising among patients already in the Institution. Hints on precautionary measures in general were given out for the benefit of the public, and with much advantage. The measures adopted in the house were effectual, and it is worthy of mention, that during the prevalence of the epidemic in the Autumn of 1849, the Infirmary was comparatively deserted, everybody outside the house appearing to shun the place in the dread that the disease already filled the Hospital.

In London the Governors of the Middlesex Hospital stoutly resisted an attempt by the Cholera Board in 1832 to admit cholera patients, for they considered that any such admission would 'place in jeopardy the lives of the patients already within the Hospital'.[28] The authorities at the Westminster Hospital also refused, but in 1848 the Medical Committee was asked to report 'on the best means to be adopted in respect of any cases that may arise of cholera'.[29] The outcome of the report was:[30]

> that in the event of epidemic cholera appearing in Westminster the Medical Committee are of the opinion that should cases be presented for admission they should be taken in the ordinary course, but in the event of cases becoming numerous that one or more wards be set apart for their reception.

The two royal hospitals of St Bartholomew's and St Thomas's admitted cholera patients to separate buildings without any discussion over the merit of such action.

As attitudes changed towards the admittance of cholera patients, so a similar move took place with regard to cases of fever. Hospitals continued to become more aware of their responsibilities. In 1830 the Birmingham General Hospital reported that 'separate Wards for the reception of infectious or offensive cases are now completed'.[31] These wards were in constant use during the outbreaks of fever and smallpox in the town and in the hospital itself. The Lincoln County Hospital converted two cottages adjoining the garden in 1840 to take infectious cases. The cottages were occupied 'by cases of Small-pox and Fever, which would necessarily, had it not been for this outlay, have occupied the same ward, if not the adjoining bed, and have been attended upon by the same nurse as their fellow patients'.[32]

At Sheffield General Infirmary:[33]

> The erection of [a] new wing called the House of Recovery, and originally designed for fever wards, was a subject that occupied the Weekly Board for several years. That building was opened in 1844, and some fever patients were admitted, but further experience showed that such cases could not be safely dealt with in a general hospital, and after some time the accommodation in that wing was made available for the ordinary purposes of the hospital.

The voluntary hospitals in Scotland appear to have had no compunction about admitting fever patients. It was considered to be part of their duty to treat such patients, and the dangers were thought to be minimal.[34]

From its opening in 1794 the Glasgow Royal Infirmary undertook the treatment of infectious fevers. In the five years following its opening:[35]

> 14 per cent. of all the admissions suffered from 'fever', and in 1816, when the accommodation had been increased to 230 beds, this was found of incalculable use as a receptacle for persons with low fever, the multitudes of whom, flocking from the closes and ill-aired alleys and lanes of the city, exceeded all precedent.

The report for 1817 commented on this outbreak of typhus fever and stated that the Directors had received 'all fever patients, without being very scrupulous about their recommendations'.[36] In December of that year the numbers who applied to be admitted became overwhelming and it was ordered that the recommenders would have to pay £3 for each patient over the number normally allowed.[37] The fever was also prevalent in Edinburgh, and the Royal Infirmary opened three additional wards, but these were not sufficient. The Managers, therefore, took over the unoccupied Queensberry House Barracks to be used as a fever hospital for sixty to eighty patients on 23 February 1818, 'trusting that the public would respond in such a way as to provide the necessary increased expenditure'.[38] The comments of the report for that year are extremely illuminating:[39]

> In consequence of the increase of fever cases, more than usual caution became necessary, in airing and cleaning the bedding; and one of the wards was in consequence fitted up, in which this operation is accomplished in a very ingenious and successful manner. . . . One of the principal Physicians was for a time affected with this fever, while seven out of ten of the clerks suffered severely, and three of these have been affected a second time. The matron and several of the nurses died of this fever caught in the Hospital, and all the nurses in the Fever Wards have suffered from it:

The sequence of events at Aberdeen has a familiar ring.[40]

> Strangely enough the city was visited in 1818 by a serious epidemic of fever, supposed to have been brought from Glasgow by a female pauper lunatic. The fever wards of the Infirmary were filled to overflowing, and the Managers were obliged to look out for a suitable building to be utilized as a temporary hospital. And to that end a large well-aired manufacturing house on the Gallowgate was placed at their disposal and opened as an hospital on 1st December 1818. But even that proved insufficient, and permission was sought and obtained to occupy, first the military hospital and then the barracks, as houses of recovery.

The Infirmary and the people of the city undoubtedly took advice from the Aberdeen Medico-Chirurgical Society, for it had been asked by the President and Managers of the Infirmary to draw up a statement 'of the progress of the present epidemic fever and what steps they considered most proper to be taken in order to prevent its increase'.[41] A handbill was drawn up and distributed in the city. It stated that:[42]

> The causes of the fever which at present prevails in this city have been found to depend, in a great measure, on want of cleanliness and ventilation, along with a crowded state of the apartments of the lower classes of the people, and to be kept

F

up and spread by improper communication between the sick and healthy. . . .

It recommended a number of public health precautions, including 'Early removal to the Infirmary or House of Recovery will be the best means of insuring the safety of the sick themselves, and of preventing the spreading of the infection to others'.[43]

This evidence suggests that the voluntary hospitals, both in England and Scotland, were becoming more humane in their attitudes towards fever. Opinion at the beginning of the nineteenth century was that fever patients should be separated from the other patients by the use of isolated wards or specially constructed fever hospitals. This opinion began to alter towards the middle of the century, as many of the medical and nursing staff of these institutions had contracted fever, and a reaction was building up in favour of mixing the fever patients with the general patients. In 1842 Dr Graham of Edinburgh corresponded with many leading physicians in London and the provinces and the opinion was unanimously in favour of mixing the fever patients, provided the proportion was kept low, rather than having separate fever wards. A survey was made in 1860 on behalf of the London Hospital; sixty-four hospitals in the United Kingdom were circulated by Dr Murchison and:[44]

Replies were received from 40: viz., from 11 in London; 20 in the provinces of England; 4 in Scotland; and 5 in Ireland. Of the 11 London Hospitals, 8 admitted a very limited number of fever-cases among the general patients, while 3, viz., University College, the London, and the Marylebone General Infirmary admitted no cases of fever. Of 20 hospitals in the provinces of England 9 refused to admit fever-patients, 6 admitted them into separate wards, and only 5 distributed them among the general patients. There were also at least 6 hospitals for the special treatment of fever in the provinces of England. In every one of the 4 Scotch hospitals (Edinburgh, Glasgow, Aberdeen, and Dundee) there were separate fever wards. (Footnote – Since 1860, an hospital specially for fever has been erected in Glasgow). In Edinburgh alone, the managers permitted two fever-beds in each of the clinical wards (of 19 beds) for the purpose of instructing the students. . . . With the exception of London, then the prevalent custom was, and still is, to isolate cases of contagious fever. The different practice in London is due partly to the desire of affording to students the opportunity

of studying cases of fever, and partly to the circumstance that
a large proportion of the fever cases admitted into the London
Hospitals are examples of enteric fever, which never spreads
in the wards like typhus. . . . But even in the London Hospitals,
it is universally admitted that there is a danger of true typhus
spreading, if the number of cases be greater than 1 in 5, or
1 in 6; so that practically, the necessity of the Fever Hospital
for the surplus, which during epidemics may be enormous, is
conceded.

The admission or exclusion of fever cases was taken up in the
report on hospitals to the Privy Council in 1864[45] for a number of
reasons:[46]

the admission of cases of infectious diseases forms a very
important item in regulating the mortality of a hospital; and
this is not merely because infectious diseases, such as typhus
and small-pox, present normally a far larger percentage
mortality than most other cases admitted into hospitals, but
because practically, the admission or non-admission of this
class of affections regulates in no small degree the admission of
other acute medical diseases. Thus, if it be the regulation of a
hospital that no cases of fever be admitted, and the regulation
be enforced, not only do actual fever cases cease to apply, but
all those cases (and they are numerous) in regard to which a
skilled medical practitioner would hesitate perhaps to commit
himself to an opinion, ceases also to apply. So that the
hospital which declines to receive fever cases into its wards,
ceases in large proportion to receive cases of acute internal
inflammation which really form the great bulk of the urgent
cases which physicians are called upon to treat.

The authors went on to compare the death-rates prevailing in those
hospitals which accepted fever cases, finding that in the London
Fever Hospital for the year 1861 the general mortality was 18·2 per
cent, while:[47]

the mortality of the 173 non-infectious cases amounted to
28·3. . . . The hospital at Stafford has a special fever department. The mortality of the whole establishment was during 1862,
7·5 %; but the percentage of deaths among the fever
cases amounted to 25; and that of all cases (exclusive of fever)
to 6 only. . . . the Glasgow Infirmary; for the year 1862 the

death-rate for the whole institution amounted to 10·3 %; but the death-rate in the fever wards was 16·7, and that of the hospital (excluding fever cases from computation) 8·7 only.

Despite the evidence produced in their own report and in other well-known contemporary writings the authors were of the opinion that cases of fever, i.e. typhus and scarlatina, could be admitted in the proportion of one to six[48] into general wards which were spacious and well ventilated. The report was criticized on this point by a number of medical authorities at the time. An anonymous writer in 1865 made the following cogent points about the admission of fever cases:[49]

> We are sure that we are within the mark in saying that during the last three years 150 patients have contracted typhus in the general hospitals of London. . . . With the evidence before us, we cannot but regard it as a most unjustifiable practice to admit patients suffering from some trifling disease, such as quinsy, rheumatism, or dyspepsia, into the wards of a general hospital, and to make them run the risk of catching typhus or scarlatina, and of thus losing their lives.

The author then compared the rate at which these diseases spread at the London Fever Hospital and at the general hospitals in London during the first six months of 1861:[50]

> The 1080 cases admitted into the Fever Hospital communicated the disease to 27 persons, of whom 8 died. . . . But the 272 cases admitted into the six general hospitals (St. Mary's, St. Bart's, St. Thomas's, Guy's, Middlesex, and the German Hospital) communicated the disease to 71 persons, of whom 21 died.

A physician to the Bristol Infirmary wrote that, though he did not approve of the practice:[51]

> there is scarcely an hospital in the kingdom of a perfect construction, perfect at least in the way of being fitted for the treatment of contagious diseases at all, [and] I am only able to agree with the report, to the extent that the treatment of such diseases might be undertaken better in general wards than in a crowded cottage.

In the provinces the only hospitals which admitted fever patients to the general wards at this time were those at Bath, Chichester, Reading and Oxford.[52]

Even in the best-regulated hospitals outbreaks of infectious disease occurred despite the improvements in diagnosis. An outbreak of smallpox, for example, occurred at St George's Hospital in 1870. It was reported that:[53]

> we have had twenty cases attacked with small-pox in the Hospital; four having received the infection in the house were discharged, and afterwards attacked with the disease; and three were admitted before the appearance of the eruption – the febrile symptoms being attributed to other causes. Of these twenty-seven cases, six died – four in, and two out of the Hospital.

Although the Sanitary Act, 1866, empowered the local Sewer Authority in the provinces and the Nuisance Authority in London to provide and maintain hospitals for infectious diseases, little was done. It was under the Metropolitan Poor Act, 1867, that in London the united Metropolitan Asylums Board started to establish such institutions. The Public Health Act, 1875, enabled local authorities to make provision for patients suffering from infectious diseases, but even at this date the hospitals had a role to play and the controversy was by no means over. The Superintendent of Guy's Hospital, writing of mortality in hospitals, commented:[54]

> It is now generally recognized that during the prevalence of epidemics in large towns, there is a positive necessity for finding separate accommodation for the disease in hospitals specifically set apart for the purpose, but it is still very doubtful whether the concentration of a large number of persons suffering from similar maladies has not an evil influence in intensifying the virulence of the disease. It is held by many, and the practice is not yet abandoned in many hospitals, that by placing one or two patients suffering from fever in a large ward with ordinary diseases, their chances of recovery are strengthened, and that the dangers from contagion are reduced to a minimum.

Thus, the debate continued, and the committee inquiring into the benefits of fever hospitals heard evidence in 1878 from Guy's, St Thomas's, the London, St Bart's, St George's, the Westminster and the Middlesex Hospitals, all of which were in favour of admitting fever cases to the general wards. This practice was, happily, no longer so prevalent as previously, as for example, with the Glasgow Royal Infirmary which had handed over responsibility for the treatment of fever cases to the local authority in 1876.

The practice with regard to the treatment of fever cases, therefore, emerges as a complex one in which generalizations are not possible. The position varied from hospital to hospital and even from year to year. Starting from a policy of complete exclusion, the general move was to acceptance in separate fever wards or in separate buildings. The practice then altered to one of admitting fever patients to the general wards in small numbers, but the potential dangers were eventually realized and the policy reverted to one of separation in buildings specifically set aside for the purpose. These institutions were normally outside the voluntary hospital system, being provided by the local authorities, particularly after the Public Health Act, 1875. Those hospitals which accepted fever patients were liable to exhibit higher rates of mortality as the likelihood of death for a patient suffering from fever was greater than for a patient suffering from other non-infectious diseases.[55]

8 Surgery

The popular notion of the practice of surgery during the eighteenth and most part of the nineteenth centuries is that it was nasty and brutish, but never short. Surgery had always had a lower status than the practice of physic as the cutting of flesh was contrary to the Hippocratic Oath. It became the province of quacks and charlatans; the main areas of treatment being the removal of cataracts, cutting for the stone and traction to remove a dislocation. At the beginning of the eighteenth century there was little formal training available for surgeons, in fact, a number of the respectable surgeons learnt and developed their techniques from the quacks. Training gradually developed through the system of apprenticeship to a practising surgeon during the second half of the eighteenth century after the connection with the barbers had been severed in 1745. The apprenticeship system itself was largely overtaken by the demands of the Apothecaries Act, 1815, which required a formal set of teaching and a period of walking the wards.[1] In 1824 it was only possible to gain recognized qualifications through the hospitals in London, Edinburgh, Aberdeen and Dublin. The position became increasingly impossible as the apprentices who went through the provincial hospitals were at a disadvantage, so in 1832 a number of anatomy schools were recognized in provincial towns which possessed voluntary hospitals. In 1843 the Royal College of Surgeons of London was reconstituted to form the Royal College of Surgeons of England, and as a result fellowship was now obtainable by examination.[2] 'Thus the status of the surgeon in England underwent a radical change between the years 1815 and 1845; during this time he developed from an ill-educated technician, trained by apprenticeship alone, into a highly qualified member of the medical profession.'[3] It is against this background of slowly developing training methods that surgical treatment in the eighteenth and nineteenth centuries must be judged. A lack of knowledge of the function and anatomy of many of the organs of the body, particularly during the eighteenth century, hampered the growth of surgery and the desire for furthering knowledge was curtailed by the relatively short supply of cadavers which could be obtained for dissection.[4] The only well-established operation which involved the exploration of an internal organ was lithotomy, i.e. the removal of a stone from the urinary bladder.[5] Abdominal operations were completely unknown except for some unsuccessful attempts at Caesarean section in hopeless cases. Prior to the introduction of anaesthesia in 1846,[6] both the scope and numbers of surgical operations were limited. The principal areas in which surgical intervention was necessary were limited to lithotomy, amputation for compound fractures and the 'white swelling' of scrofula, the setting of simple fractures, operation for cataract, trephining of the skull for depressed fractures and meningeal haemorrhage, incision of abscesses and carbuncles including the draining of 'psoas abscess' (another tubercular complaint) and the removal of cysts.

Operations were considered to be special events and none could be carried out until a set procedure had been observed – 'That no Amputation, or other great Operation, except an urgent Occasion require it, be performed without a previous Consultation of the Physicians and Surgeons'.[7] In the days prior to the use of anaesthesia surgeons were loath to operate because of the great pain which would be caused and the shock to the body.[8] 'In pre-anaesthetic days operations were rushed through at lightning speed and under conditions of appalling difficulty. The most hardened surgeons had to steel themselves to perform operations which they knew would cause agony to their patients and nerve-racking distress to themselves.'[9] Perhaps the speed necessary to perform a surgical operation encouraged greater skill on the part of the surgeon and minimized the shock to the patient.

Of the 960 admissions to the Worcester General Infirmary during the thirty-three months from its opening, only 10 surgical operations were recorded: 'Five Amputations of the Leg were performed – Two Cancerous Breasts extirpated; Two Cataracts depressed; and One Boy cut for the Stone, with the desired success'.[10]

In the period from 8 December 1794 to 1 January 1796 the surgeons of the Glasgow Royal Infirmary undertook 32 principal operations, this number being out of a total of 276 in-patients admitted during this time; while in 1800 of 803 in-patients admitted, 41 underwent surgery. Unfortunately the results of the operations were not published, though the main items listed were the familiar ones of amputations, repairs of fistulas, extirpation of cancers and tapping[11] – a very limited field of surgery.

A later survey of the surgical practice at the Liverpool Infirmary between 1821 and 1843 concentrated on the same operations with the addition of the ligaturing of aneurisms which had been introduced in the early years of the nineteenth century. The heaviest mortality was recorded for operations on hernias, and the partial removal of bones in cases of compound fractures, particularly in the thigh and humerus – in these cases the death-rate reaches 25 per cent. The safest surgery recorded at a figure of one death in thirty-six cases was amputation of the hand or foot.[12] This list can be compared with the number and results of operations performed at the same hospital in the mid-1830s, when from the total of 43 patients who suffered amputations only 3 died, and of 37 other operations only 6 were fatal. The two lists were comparable in the death-rates recorded, though, it is possible that the years 1834, 1835 and 1836 were particularly successful.[13]

Details of individual operations have not generally survived, but a notebook has come to light of the operations performed at the General Infirmary at Leeds for the early 1820s.[14] Fifty-two operations had been recorded ranging from amputation to couching of the eye. On 13 May 1823 Mr Hey operated on James Fearnley, aged twenty-one, and the observer reported that 'Three separate hard tumours removed from left Mamma – No inflammation followed – Wound healed in patient by 1st intention, in patient by suppuration and granulation; Two or Three deepish Abscesses formed during progress of case requiring Scalpel – little or no Constitutional disturbance'. An 'Amputation of Thigh for White Swelling of Knee Joint' was performed by Mr Hey on Mary Masterman, aged nine, on 3 June 1823. Apparently, she 'did well'. On the nineteenth of the same month Mr Chorley performed a lithotomy operation on Duncan Mackrile – 'upwards of 100 Stones were extracted several of which had the Appearance of having been previously united – Operation lasted 1⅓ Hours'.[15] The last operation recorded was for 1 August 1824 when Mr Hey performed a 'Couching of right Eye' on Jos. Pace.

It would appear reasonable that the scope and numbers of surgical operations remained limited during the early years of the nineteenth century, because of the pain to the patient and the incomplete knowledge of the anatomy of the human body. The hospitals did not in general publish any information on operations performed, and as the historian of the Manchester Infirmary noted:[16]

It is curious that throughout all these years there is no indication of the number of operations that were taking place. However, in 1833 the Board requested the house-surgeons to produce a statement of the number of operations performed by each surgeon during the last two years. The statement is most interesting. In that period Mr John Thorp had operated on five occasions only, Mr Ransome, on fifteen, Mr Ainsworth on twelve, Mr Robert Thorpe on fifteen, Mr Wilson on twenty-seven and Mr Turner on twenty.

The committee of the House of Commons which reported on medical education in 1834 requested information from the voluntary hospitals on all aspects of their work, including details of operations performed. The return of the Edinburgh Royal Infirmary disclosed that 31 capital operations were undertaken from 1 October 1830 to 1 October 1831, 15 in 1831–2, 38 in 1832–3, and 63 in 1833–4.[17] Thus, again the small number of operations is noticeable at a time when the Infirmary was admitting approximately 3,000 in-patients annually, of which surgical patients represented about one-third.

The surgeons of the provincial voluntary hospitals in the market towns operated even less frequently. For instance, at the Salisbury General Infirmary 'there were about six operations a year recorded in the operations book – most of the surgery being carried out for injury, tuberculosis, or bladder stone'.[18] In 1838 the only operations recorded were two amputations at the thigh, one lithotomy and one removal of a testicle.

Anaesthesia

The first great breakthrough in the practice of surgery came with the introduction and general acceptance of anaesthetic measures.:[19]

> [The] philosophy of bottom (q.v.), did more to delay the introduction of anaesthesia than anything else. . . . A change in Man's attitude towards suffering in general was necessary before his attention would be directed towards the pain of surgery in particular. Thus the introduction of anaesthesia is a dramatic outward expression of Man's inner change from eighteenth-century brutality to our own more humane pattern of behaviour.

Knowledge about the use of anaesthetics had been available for many years, as alcohol and opium had been used for centuries, but an effective dose of opium would have to be dangerously large and the obvious pain-killer of alcohol was infrequently used by the respectable surgeon in a good practice.

The account of the first use of ether as an anaesthetic is too well known for a detailed report to be given here; suffice to say that it was first administered on 16 October 1846 by Thomas Morton in the Massachusetts General Hospital for the dissection of a tuberculous gland in the neck of a young man. Though this technique was used in private in London and possibly at the Dumfries and Galloway Royal Infirmary on or about 17 December 1846,[20] the first operation under the influence of ether of any significance in the United Kingdom was the amputation of a leg on 21 December 1846 by Robert Liston of University College Hospital. 'The acceptance of ether by the leading surgeon of London did more to introduce anaesthesia into England than any "first" administration.'[21] From this small start the surgeons of the voluntary hospitals soon took up the idea of anaesthesia, first in London, and then in the provinces. The provincial hospitals were not slow in adopting the technique, thus, for instance, ether was administered at the Northampton General Hospital on 28 January 1847, only six weeks after the demonstration by Robert Liston in London.[22]

However, ether was not the ideal anaesthetic agent, and chloroform was substituted in the closing months of 1847 after experiments by J. Y. Simpson:[23]

> During the last week the chloroform has been employed as a means of allaying pain during surgical operations in most London hospitals. As far as we can learn, the result of this experiment, as tested in several capital operations, has been to show that this agent produces its effect with more rapidity and certainty than the vapour of ether, and that its action appears to be attended with fewer disagreeable consequences – such as the evidences of pulmonary irritation, &c. Its influence as regards the condition of the patient during the operation is considered to be nearly identical with that of ether.

The Governors of the Newcastle Infirmary in their report for 1849–50 noted with gratification:[24]

> after the painful contemplation of such an amount of human suffering, as the list of operations presents, that to learn that in all of them, and in many other equally painful cases, the soporific effect of chloroform have always blessed the sufferers

with happy oblivion of their woes, and often substituted, in the place of excruciating pain, dreams of happier, bygone times.

Chloroform, like ether, was a dangerous drug and had to be administered with care. However, the dangers were not fully recognized and the quantities given were not regulated; and its administration was often entrusted to a servant who was not qualified. As a result deaths did occur from its maladministration, the first being recorded as taking place near Newcastle on 28 January 1848 – Hannah Greener, aged fifteen, died under an anaesthetic for the removal of a toe-nail, and from the evidence available it would appear that the patient died from an overdose of chloroform causing paralysis of the heart.

Considerable controversy attended the introduction of anaesthetic techniques, particularly over the use of chloroform, and the effects on surgical mortality. However, it should be borne in mind that, though at first there was no change at least in the type of surgery performed, as time went on and experience was gained surgeons began to take advantage of the prolonged time in which a patient could be safely kept under the influence of anaesthesia to develop new surgical techniques and operations. The surgeon to the Salisbury General Infirmary made an analysis of the situation prior to and after the introduction of anaesthesia to answer some of the more vociferous criticisms of the use of chloroform:[25]

> In some ingenious and well written papers, Dr. James Arnott has sought to prove that Chloroform is not only immediately dangerous in operations; but that it renders the subsequent progress of the patients less satisfactory than when they were performed without it: and he has published tables to prove the mortality since the introduction of this anaesthetic, to have increased from 21 to 34 per cent. . . . He drew up his tables from data, taken from the books of the largest and most celebrated London Hospitals, extending for each era over three years. I have extended my tables over six years previous to, and six years after the introduction of Chloroform, leaving out the intermediate twelve months; as during that interval some patients were submitted to anaesthetics, some were not; again, in some, sulphuric ether was used, others, Chloroform.

Of 31 amputations of the thigh, leg and arm performed at the Salisbury General Infirmary between 1 January 1841 and 31 December 1846, 7 terminated fatally. In the period from 1 January

1849 to 31 December 1855 54 amputations were carried out, of which 5 were fatal. 'So that whereas we lost in the six years previous to the use of Chloroform, 22·58 per cent we had a mortality of only 9·259 per cent during the six years following its introduction.'[26] The writer found that previous to the introduction of chloroform the mortality-rates in the London hospitals and the Salisbury General Infirmary had been very similar at 21 per cent and 22 per cent, respectively, and that the great difference after the introduction of the anaesthetic agent could be explained by the different methods of administration. In the London hospitals the chloroform was given on a cloth, while at the Salisbury General Infirmary it was administered through a Snow's inhaler which regulated the amount being given to the patient.

The small difference in the types of operations performed in the years immediately after the introduction of anaesthesia can be seen in a report of the Newcastle Infirmary:[27]

Irrespective of the numerous small operations performed during the course of the treatment of the surgical cases and accidents, and of the number of dislocations and fractures set and reduced, which amounted to upwards of 240, the following operations have been performed during the year:—Of amputations of limbs there have been 13, of portions of limbs 23, of other parts of the body 15, of tumours 14, operations for lithotomy 1 (which is an unusually small number), on diseased bones 12, for hydrocele 14, for fistula 6, arteries tied 4, and on 13 deformities from contractions of tendons, or of the skin after the healing of burns. With the exception of two deaths from amputations, all the other operations have been perfectly successful.

A survey made of the operations performed in 117 hospitals in England and Wales in the year 1863 indicated that of 3,440 performed only 290 were fatal, a death-rate of 8·43 per cent.[28] However, if the 1,122 operations about the eye were excluded from this figure the death-rate rises to 12·51 per cent; though this corrected figure is not completely accurate, for if the death-rate of the 1,371 principal operations where 210 deaths were recorded is calculated the final figure rises further to 15·3 per cent. The number of operations performed of specific types and the deaths recorded for each throws some light on the controversy which raged about surgical mortality after the introduction of anaesthesia. Ovariotomy, the removal of an ovarian cyst, was an operation which had hitherto only been performed on the rarest occasion, but was now within the scope of general surgery because of the extra time which anaesthesia made available. However, its success was not overwhelming, though it was not performed very frequently. Of 22 cases recorded in 1863, only 5 were classified as being cured or relieved, thus giving a death-rate of 77·27 per cent. Other explorations of the anatomy, for example for paracentesis of the abdomen, thorax and bladder, also recorded high death-rates. Twelve deaths were registered from 38 operations of this type recorded, giving a death-rate of 31·58 per cent. Surgical mortality at individual hospitals varied considerably, a partial explanation being the differing methods of calculation.[29] The Norfolk and Norwich Hospital recorded a death-rate of 4·56 per cent on the 302 operations which its surgeons performed in 1863, but this figure included 105 'minor operations'. The highest surgical death-rate registered was for St Bartholomew's Hospital where 429 operations were performed on 417 patients of which 64 died, giving a figure of 14·91 per cent, while the General Infirmary at Leeds followed closely behind recording a death-rate of 13·02 per cent. The surgical mortality for the other hospitals fluctuated between the low of 2·02 per cent claimed by the Salisbury General Infirmary and the 10·05 per cent of the Southern Hospital, Liverpool. The average surgical mortality of the eleven hospitals listed was 6·71 per cent.[30]

The figures given may appear high by present-day standards, though some are extremely low, but they are considerably lower than some would have the historian to believe. Further, it may be noted that 'it is the overall surgical mortality that matters; a patient is just as dead whether death is caused by operation or by failure to operate; anaesthesia, by making operation possible, reduced the death rate'.[31] The principal source of death, after anaesthesia had removed the shock, was sepsis, and it needed the breakthrough of Lister's antiseptic principles, first used in 1865, to alter materially surgical mortality.[32]

The scope of surgical techniques widened continually with the ability of the surgeon to explore and examine all parts of the anatomy of the body. As an illustration, the principal operations at the General Infirmary at Leeds in 1860 were classified under 43 headings, and in this year of 179 operations performed, 147 were claimed to have cured the patients, 20 relieved, and 12 patients died.[33] In 1875 the classification of the principal operations performed had been extended to 108 headings, though this did not reflect the breakdown of individual operations. Thus, for instance, the removal of tumours was divided into 16 subsections, depending upon the type of tumour operated on. Six hundred and sixteen operations were performed in this year, more than three times the number of 1860, from which 39 died, 45 were relieved and 532 were cured.[34] Some of the more interesting operations which emerge from the list are two successful colostomies, the making of a false anus when the lower part of the large bowel is obstructed; seven ovariotomies, of which only two were successful; and a claimed successful operation on a patient with spina bifida.

Thus, by 1875 surgical practice was developing into the science which was to make great strides forward during the period to the First World War. This development was certainly not foreseen by many surgeons of the day, as witness a definitive statement by one of them, J. E. Erichsen, to University College Hospital in 1873:[35]

> That there must be a final limit to development in this
> department of our profession there can be no doubt. The art of
> surgery is but the application of manipulative methods to the
> relief and cure of injury and disease. Like every other art, be it
> manipulative, plastic, or imitative, it can only be carried to a
> certain definite point of excellence. An art may be modified, it
> may be varied, but it cannot be perfected beyond certain
> attainable limits. And so it is, and indeed must be, with
> surgery. There cannot always be fresh fields for conquest by
> the knife: there must be portions of the human frame that will
> ever remain sacred from its intrusion, at least in the surgeon's
> hands. That we have nearly, if not quite, reached these final
> limits, there can be little question.

A remark of singularly false prophecy in the light of what was to come.

To understand more fully the role of surgery in the eighteenth and nineteenth centuries it would be worth while to examine three of the principal operations in greater detail, namely, amputation, lithotomy and lithotrity, and herniotomy.

Amputation

> The frequency of its performance, the mutilation which it
> causes, its severity, and its immediate and ultimate dangers,
> combine in making the operation of amputation one of the

most important subjects which can occupy the attention of the practical and operative surgeon. . . . In private practice, in the better ranks of society, it is an operation of comparatively rare performance; whereas in hospitals it exceeds many fold all the other capital operations.[36]

Amputation is an old-established practice, owing its skill in performance to the wounds of wars and battles. In civil practice amputation was usually carried out for injury, which is self-evident, or for disease, commonly of a tubercular origin – 'white swellings', 'strumous', 'scrophulous', etc. – or because of a bone deficiency – 'caries'.[37]

The performance of amputation has never enjoyed a good reputation, but it should be remembered that variations in the death-rate occur according to the limb to be amputated and the cause of the amputation. The general view expressed is that 'in 1800 40 to 50 per cent of patients died under surgical operations'.[38] This figure would appear to have no foundation when the figures for the nineteenth century are examined, for unless there was some sudden improvement in technique, the records from the nineteenth century suggest an entirely contrary opinion. Over a period of twenty-two years from 1821 the death-rate recorded at the Liverpool Infirmary averaged one in six for amputation of the leg, one in eleven for the thigh, one in eighteen for the arm, and one in thirty-six for the hand or foot.[39] However, these claimed figures do appear very low when compared with those given for the surgical practice at the Glasgow Royal Infirmary for the years from 1795 to 1838. In 72 cases of amputation the overall death-rate was 51·3 per cent, varying from 91·6 per cent in 12 cases of amputation of the thigh, to complete success in 15 cases of the removal of the forearm.[40] A survey made of the surgical operations performed in the London hospitals from 1840 to 1841 showed that 117 amputations were successfully completed, while 69 were fatal.[41] The surgeon to the Devon and Exeter Hospital was able to collect from the notes of cases a total of 300 amputations performed between 1816 and 1849. Of 68 primary and intermediate amputations, 18 were fatal – 15 of these were of the leg or thigh; of secondary and intermediate, 7 were fatal out of 26 performed; and of 206 for disease, only 18 died.[42]

The number of cases of amputation in the University College Hospital, from the last day of June 1835, to the termination of the year 1840, a period of six years and a half, has been 66, and of these, 56 have proved successful, while 10 have been attended with fatal results, at a variable period of time after the performance of the operation.[43]

A later report of the amputations performed by one of the surgeons to St Thomas's Hospital between 1835 and 1840 showed that 13 died out of 54 operated upon. The surgeon wrote that:[44]

> putting these together with the cases at University College Hospital, it must be evident, that the mortality is a long way below the 50 to 75 per cent which has been stated, by some surgical writers, as the ordinary average of fatal amputations. It will be observed also that the largest mortality is among the cases operated on for accidents, and on the lower extremities. In 7 amputations through the thigh, I lost 6; and of 9 through the leg, 3 died. Whilst of 6 primary and 1 secondary amputations in the upper extremity, not a single case was lost. This excess of mortality in operating after accidents, is to be ascribed, when the patients die early, to the conjoined shock of the accident and operation. Besides which the persons admitted into hospitals for such injuries are commonly free livers with broken down constitutions, the like of whom are not unfrequently destroyed by the results of trivial accidents, which run either into erysipelas, or diffuse cellular inflammation and gangrene.

Taking the period covering the introduction of anaesthesia from 1839 to 1849 at the Glasgow Royal Infirmary, from 169 amputations performed there were 62 deaths which gave an improved death-rate of 36·6 per cent when compared with 1795 to 1838.[45]

The Radcliffe Infirmary, Oxford, started an operations book in 1838,[46] which was believed to be 'a faithful record of the higher operations performed in the house from that time':[47]

> Of the 89 amputations for disease, 82 are recorded as for diseases of joints; they are mostly described as being of strumous character. . . . Of other disease, not of strumous character, under the names of caries, necrosis, cancer or cancerous, gangrene, and elephantiasis, 7 are recorded. . . . Of the 89 patients who underwent amputation for disease, ten died, – one after removal of the leg, and nine after that of the thigh.

All of the five patients who underwent secondary amputations for accident recovered.

G

The controversy surrounding the effect of anaesthesia on surgical mortality resulted in a committee being established by the Royal Medical and Chirurgical Society in 1864 to inquire into the available published statistics on mortality after amputation. The results of the study were not in any way firmly conclusive as to the effects of anaesthesia, tending to suggest that the mortality after amputation did not materially alter. A death-rate of 20·1 per cent on 1,213 amputations for disease was recorded in the London and provincial hospitals for the period prior to the use of anaesthesia, and for amputations in respect of accident the death-rate was 39·5 per cent on 889 cases reported. This gave an overall mortality-rate of 27·4 per cent prior to its use. Subsequent to the introduction of anaesthesia on figures published to 1864, the death-rates were 22·0 per cent on 1,154 cases for disease, 33·9 per cent on 668 cases for accident, which gave an overall figure for mortality of 26·1 per cent; a fall of 1·3 per cent on the preceding years.[48] In the report to the Privy Council in 1864 on the state of hospitals the authors attempted a survey of operations and their results, the tables being constructed from material available for varying lengths of time in different hospitals. It is noticeable again that the rates of mortality varied according to the type of amputation, and to a certain extent on where the amputation was performed. The highest figure recorded was 36·0 per cent for amputation of the thigh at the hip in 158 cases in London hospitals, and the lowest was 7·63 per cent for amputation of the forearm in 118 cases in large provincial towns:[49]

> But the list is, unfortunately, notwithstanding that we have taken considerable pains in collecting the statistics, very imperfect. The actual causes of death have been furnished to us for a very small proportion only of the total number of cases, and the distinction between amputation for injury and amputation for disease has very frequently indeed not been made.

For the year 1863 only it was found that of 567 unspecified amputations performed in the hospitals of England and Wales in that year 482 were claimed to cure or relieve and only 85 were fatal, giving a mortality-rate of 14·99 per cent.[50] In contrast, between 1835 and 1865 at the Dumfries and Galloway Royal Infirmary 59 amputations were performed with 13 deaths – a death-rate of 22·03 per cent – but 8 of these deaths were as a result of amputation of the thigh which exhibited a death-rate of 30·7 per cent.[51]

It was not until December 1852 that the surgeons of the General Infirmary at Leeds started to register the operations performed in that hospital. The numbers have been tabulated to May 1869 when the Old Infirmary was closed:[52]

out of 111 operations in which (excluding the minor operations) the whole or a considerable part of the hand was removed, 108 recovered and only 3 died, being 36 recoveries to 1 death; out of 81 amputations of the forearm, there were 74 recoveries to 7 deaths, or $10\frac{1}{2}$ recoveries to each death; of 82 upper arm amputations, 59 recovered and 23 died, being rather more than $2\frac{1}{2}$ recoveries to each death; of 11 shoulder amputations, 6 recovered, while 5 died, or $1\frac{1}{5}$ recoveries to 1 death. Of 68 foot amputations (excluding the minor), 61 recovered and 7 died, or nearly 9 recoveries to each death; of 10 recorded (there must have been more) ankle-joint amputations, 9 recovered and 1 died; of 168 amputations of the leg, 125 recovered and 43 died, being nearly 3 recoveries to each fatal case; of 107 amputations in the lower or middle thigh, 74 recovered and 33 died, being nearly $2\frac{1}{4}$ recoveries to 1 death; of 18 upper thigh amputations, 9 recovered and 9 died; and of 2 amputations at the hip-joint, 1 recovered and one died. Thus it will be seen that not only is the mortality greater in proportion to the size of the part of an extremity removed, but that it is also greater for each of the corresponding portions of the lower extremity than it is for those of the upper extremity.

The evidence suggests, therefore, that the number of amputations performed was small and that the resultant mortality figures may look far worse than they could be because of the numbers involved. Thus, at St Bartholomew's Hospital between 1866 and 1875, from 392 amputations performed, there were 74 deaths, a mortality-rate of $18 \cdot 88$ per cent; but if individual cases are taken the figure varies enormously, even from one year to another. The death-rate for primary amputations averaged $18 \cdot 31$ per cent, for secondary amputations $21 \cdot 95$ per cent and for amputations for disease $18 \cdot 21$ per cent.[53]

Thus, to make any assessment of the practice of amputation, it is necessary to discern between the various categories of amputation. Mortality was undoubtedly high for some forms of amputation, particularly that of the thigh, but was very low for some others, for example, that of the arm. Therefore, before issuing a general condemnation of the practice of amputation, the evidence should be examined a little more closely to determine the nature of the amputation.[54]

Lithotomy

'I will not cut persons labouring under the stone, but will leave this to be done by men who are practitioners of this work' (Hippocratic Oath).[55]

The practice of lithotomy, like amputation, came under considerable scrutiny in the literature of the nineteenth century, as it was one of the few established and more common types of surgical operation:[56]

It is reported of Hippocrates, that he required of his pupils to abstain from the practice of lithotomy; from whence it is probable that, even in those early times, there were professed lithotomists, and from that period to the present, the lithotomist, in some measure, still holds his ground – at times; itinerant and strictly empirical, and, though brought within the pale of the profession, always affecting mystery and concealment of method; and, above all, persevering in endeavours to prove that his operations are uniformly successful.

This seemingly cynical opinion is probably nearer the truth than may at first be suspected. Lithotomy had started as a practice outside the province of the surgeon, and in England it needed William Cheselden in the early part of the eighteenth century to bring respectability to those who performed the operation. He adapted the lateral method of operation which had been introduced by Frère Jacques, a Franciscan lay-brother, and was remarkably successful. Cheselden wrote:[57]

what success I have had in my private practice I have kept no account of, because I had not intention to publish it, that not being sufficiently witnessed. Publickly in St Thomas's Hospital I have cut two hundred and thirteen; of the first fifty only three died; of the second fifty, three; of the third fifty, eight, and of the last sixty-three, six. Several of these patients had the small pox during their cure, some of which died, but I think not more in proportion that what usually die of that distemper; these are not reckon'd among those who died of the operation. The

reason why so few died in the two first fifties was, at that time
few very bad cases offered; in the third, the operation being in
high request, even the most aged and most miserable cases
expected to be sav'd by it; besides, at that time, I made the
operation lower in hopes of improving it; but found I was
mistaken.

Previous to the use of the lateral technique Cheselden had lost one
in ten, and in the high operation one in seven.

It would appear that the frequency of stone in the urinary bladder
differed considerably from one part of the country to the other. For
example, in Herefordshire it was unknown, for in the period from
the opening of the Hereford General Hospital in 1755 to 1820 'there
has not been a single applicant with stone, although there have
passed the books, 16,248 patients'.[58] At the General Infirmary at
Leeds cases of stone were not unknown, but cannot be described as
frequent. From its opening in 1767 to September 1817, 76,386
patients had been treated in the Infirmary, but of these only 197
were cut for the stone; 28 died as a result of the operation, and a
further 65 would not submit themselves to the rigours of its
performance.[59] In Scotland the operation was not performed very
frequently for the surgeons of the Edinburgh Royal Infirmary
operated on 'about 3 or 4 in as many years',[60] and the Royal
Infirmary in Aberdeen claimed 'in the last 5 years 10 operations'.[61]
To substantiate the impression that stone in the urinary bladder was
variable [in its frequency further evidence is available in the work
of one of the physicians to Guy's Hospital. In 1817 he remarked
that:[62]

In Dr. Dobson's 'Commentary on fixed Air', published in 1779,
I find a curious statistical enquiry into the different frequency
of the stone in various parts of England, from which it appears
amongst other singular results, that the proportion of calculous
cases, in the Norwich Infirmary, up to that period, was about
30 times as great as in the Cambridge Hospital. On the other
hand, he found the disease, in other parts of England,
remarkably uniform in its frequency. Thus in the Gloucester,
Worcester, Hereford, and Exeter Hospitals, the proportion of
stone cases, was 1 in 394 patients. In the North-east part of
England, including the hospitals of Newcastle, York, Leeds,
and Manchester, the proportion was 1 in 420. But in the north-
west part of England, comprehending the hospitals of Liverpool,

Chester, Shrewsbury, and the whole of North Wales, the proportion was only 1 in 3223.

The comment on the Norfolk and Norwich Hospital is most interesting as this institution gained a reputation for the performance of lithotomy. At the time the cause of the great incidence of stone in the bladder in the area around Norwich was unknown: 'The disease is almost exclusively confined to the poor; and it appears frequently in infants, before diet can have much influence. The food of our poor is by no means bad, or sparing, and the people are generally remarkable for cleanliness.'[63] The figures available for the performance of lithotomy at the Norfolk and Norwich Hospital are generally considered to be accurate, as Marcet wrote in 1817: 'All the calculi which have been extracted by operation in that hospital for the last 44 years, amounting 506, have been carefully preserved, with the circumstances annexed to each stone, and the event of the operation distinctly recorded.'[64] In these operations, a total of 70 deaths occurred, 57 of them being accounted for in the 271 adults operated upon. A senior surgeon at the Norfolk and Norwich Hospital commenting on these figures agreed that the average mortality obtained was correct, but that the failure-rate between individual surgeons was liable to fluctuation. The range was between 1 in 5¼ and 1 in 10, and he remarked that he himself 'was not very successful'[65] in the first years of his practice. By 1828, 649 cases had been operated on, of which 89 died, giving a death-rate of 1 in 7·29.[66]

But it is creditable to the state of modern surgery, and to the skill of the present surgeons of that Hospital, that in the operations performed by them (which amount to near one-third of the whole number from the commencement), the proportion of deaths has been reduced to 1 in 8·42.

Again, the size of the stone is commented upon:[67]

The operation of lithotomy is always attended with more danger, when calculi are large, than when they are small. This has been strikingly exemplified at Norwich; for of 52 cases of adult males, in which calculi of 2 oz. or more occurred, 31 died, or nearly 2 in 3; while in 282 cases, also of adult males, in which the stones weighed less than 2 oz. the mortality only amounted to 37, or rather less than 1 in 7.

The surgeons of the Glasgow Royal Infirmary operated on 15 cases between 1829 and 1832 with 2 deaths, a mortality-rate of 13·3 per cent;[68] while between the years 1844 and 1849 there were 3 deaths in the 30 cases operated on, giving a death-rate of 10·0 per cent.[69]

Between 1838 and 1853 at the Radcliffe Infirmary, Oxford, 'Of lithotomy, 33 cases are recorded in the male subject, and 4 in females. Of the male patients, 6 died'.[70] There was also one case where a calculus was found in a pouch connected to the urethra, and though the patient was claimed to be cured after the operation he suffered from incontinency as a result. 'Of the 4 cases in the female subject, none died; but it is recorded that one of them, that when discharged, 5 weeks after the operation she had not recovered the power of retaining her urine.'[71]

In all the London hospitals during the years 1840 and 1841 29 cases of the performance of lithotomy were recorded as being 'recovered' and 3 as 'fatal'.[72]

A later survey of thirteen London hospitals from January 1854 to July 1857 with regard to their practices concerning lithotomy revealed that:[73]

during the three years and a half over which our statistical Reports extended, 186 cases of lithotomy were recorded as occurring in the different Metropolitan Hospitals. It thus appears that an average of 40 patients a year are operated on for stone in the bladder. . . . This number, seeing that our list comprises thirteen Hospitals, several of them large ones, is certainly smaller than might have been expected. The modern practice of crushing has no doubt rendered this number somewhat smaller than it would otherwise have been. . . . Of the 186 cases, 146 resulted in recovery, and 40 ended in death. Of the whole number, 137 were under the age of 20, and of these 123 recovered and only 14 died; while of the 49 in which the patients were adults, we find but 23 recovered, and no fewer than 26 died. These figures show in a very strong light the influence of the age of the patient upon the prospects of a lithotomy operation. . . . There can be no doubt that the appalling mortality in patients of advanced age is in part produced by the fact that of late years the best subjects have been treated by lithotrity, and that, in the hands of many Surgeons, only those patients not considered to be in sufficiently good health to bear the latter have been submitted to lithotomy. . . . The explanation of this comparative freedom from risk in young patients, is to be found in the fact that disease of the kidneys is a very common concomitant of vesical calculus in grown-up persons, and a very rare one in children.

The overall mortality of Guy's Hospital for the performance of lithotomy over twenty-five years before 1862 was recorded as being 1 in 21½ on 230 cases. 'With five exceptions, the whole of these have been operated upon by the lateral method. In four of the five the median operation was performed, one of which died. In one the stone was extracted through the rectum.'[74]

In 1863, 80 cases of lithotomy were recorded in 117 hospitals in England and Wales, of which 10 were fatal, a death-rate of 12·5 per cent.[75]

A comprehensive list of lithotomy cases was collected in an attempt to even out the discrepancies in the analyses of operations so far presented, in so far as they were reliant on compilations and erroneous returns.[76]

This has been alluded to by Mr Henry Thompson, who has attempted to lay before the profession a more correct table, and this table may be used as a tolerably complete epitome of the mortality of lithotomy under the British Surgeons: it is derived from reliable sources, mentioned in the text of his work, (On Practical Lithotomy and Lithotrity) and contains 1827 cases.

These cases were taken from three London and six provincial hospitals and 229 deaths were recorded, giving a mortality of nearly 1 in 8.

In the report of Dr Bristowe and Mr Holmes on the state of hospitals in 1863 it was found 'that the difference between town and country hospitals is, as regards the mortality of this operation, purely trivial'.[77] A report of 1868 stated that: 'In the valuable statistical returns of St. Bartholomew's, now annually published, Mr. Willett gives a rather high death rate after lithotomy between the years 1863 and 1867.'[78] Of 48 cases, 9 were fatal, a mortality of 18·75 per cent.

At the General Infirmary at Leeds between December 1852 and May 1869, 'Of the 112 lithotomy operations, 98 recovered, and 14 died: equal to 7 recoveries to 1 death, or 1 death in every 8 cases'.[79]

Lithotrity

Thus lithotomy, though a comparatively frequent operation, could also be a dangerous one. The rectum could be wounded, the peritoneum could be opened, or a haemorrhage could be started which became difficult to stop. As a result of these dangers, instead of an open operation which involved an incision, a method was investigated of crushing the stone(s) by means of an instrument passed through the natural passage. This was a nineteenth-century development which, although having a number of advocates, was never as popular as lithotomy. A critic of the practice, writing in 1831, when lithotrity was first being popularized, stated that it was in no way preferable to lithotomy:[80]

taking into account the length of time the patient was exposed to suffering of the most severe description at each application of the instrument, (for every one must be aware that it cannot be finished at one attempt, but requires sometimes so many as seven or eight), the violent attacks of inflammation that follow it, and the weakened and exhausted state in which these attacks too frequently left the patient, so as often to render his dismissal from the hospital absolutely necessary; and even sometimes causing death itself.

Between January 1854 and July 1857, 21 patients underwent lithotrity operations in 13 London hospitals:[81]

In fifteen cases the patients were in good general health, in three the health was impaired, without being so much as to introduce any unusual degree of risk; whilst in three the patients were so ill that lithotomy was deemed to be strongly contra-indicated, and crushing was adopted as being the milder measure. . . . Of the twenty-one patients, we find that twelve recovered, that seven died, that one declined any further treatment and left the Hospital unrelieved, whilst of the remaining one the result is not known.

Benjamin Brodie, on the evidence of 9 cases of lithotrity which he had performed, found that 'the proportion of deaths to recoveries is somewhat less than 1 in $12\frac{1}{2}$' and concluded that it was safer than almost any other capital operation.[82] However, it could be argued that this was hardly a sufficiently large sample on which to base such a conclusion. As an illustration, at the General Infirmary at Leeds in the period from December 1852 to May 1869, 'Of the 25 lithotrity cases, 20 recovered, and 5 died: equal to 1 death to 4 recoveries, or 1 in 5'.[83] Thus, the practice at Leeds resulted in a death-rate more than three times that of Brodie, though the author does state:[84]

> that this record ought not to be used for the purpose of comparison with other returns of lithotrity, nor for contrasting the results of it with lithotomy, inasmuch as the greater number of deaths occurred when the operation was first practiced in the Infirmary. The later operations have been much more successful than the earlier were.

In 1868 it was remarked:[85]

> That the dangers from lithotrity are not wholly imaginary may be inferred from the statistics of the Hospital [i.e. St Bartholomew's]. It appears that the mortality from this operation is as high as 33·33 per cent, while from lithotomy it is only 18·72. But here we must correct an error, for if the young under 20 years are withdrawn the mortality after lithotomy is often about 50 per cent.

But lithotrity was never performed as frequently as lithotomy, and even this operation was not carried out in great numbers. For example, in the London hospitals in 1862 and 1863, 177 patients with stone in the bladder were admitted, 86 children and 91 adults. Of the 91 adults, only 32 were treated by lithotrity and 6 underwent no operation at all; all the children were cut for the stone.[86]

Further methods of removing stone(s) from the urinary bladder were initiated, and these operations were developed into techniques for treatment of the ureters and kidneys. Lithotomy deserves a place as one of the forerunners of modern surgery.

Herniotomy

The technique of the repair of a hernia is again a nineteenth-century innovation:[87]

> the operation was not often attempted until after the introduction of anaesthesia, except as a life saving measure for strangulation. When these early surgeons tried to deal with the ordinary hernia (which they called 'reducible' hernia because the contents of the sac could be easily pushed back into the abdominal cavity) they used the method known as herniotomy,

the simple removal of the sac without reinforcement or strengthening of the overlying wall.

The first attempts at strengthening were made by plugging the internal abdominal ring, but it was not until 1860 that methods were introduced to strengthen the tissues over the hernia. The surgeons 'reinforced the muscles with hemp string or wire sutures, materials which are not absorbed by the tissues, or they fastened pins through the muscles and interwove thread or wire from pin to pin'.[88]

At Glasgow Royal Infirmary, despite the advances in surgical technique, mortality remained high throughout the nineteenth century. Four out of 8 cases died in the period between 1829 and 1832; 6 out of 14 between 1844 and 1849; and 36 out of 73 between 1871 and 1876.[89]

The death-rate at the Radcliffe Infirmary, Oxford, was very similar to that at the Glasgow Royal Infirmary. In the operations book no record is given of any surgical treatment of a hernia before 1840 – 'Twenty-four cases of operation for strangulated hernia are recorded, beginning with the year 1840 (to 1853), in ten of which the patients died.'[90] Information is not given on the site of the hernia, but the method of treatment illustrates the primitive state of this surgery of repair – 'It was the custom upon the admission of the patient to put him at once into a hot bath, and to apply the taxis there. . . . In all the operations, the peritoneal sac was opened before the stricture was divided.'[91]

The Medical Society of Observation in its survey of the operations performed in London hospitals during 1840 and 1841 found that a total of 164 patients with strangulated hernia were admitted in these years. From this total, 91 recovered and 73 died, giving a death-rate of approximately 45 per cent.[92]

Throughout England and Wales in 1863, when the new method of surgery was in use, 567 operations were performed on patients with hernias, of which 482 were cured or relieved and 44 died, a death-rate of 26·03 per cent.[93] J. S. Bristowe and T. Holmes in their survey found that the mortality figures were consistent throughout the hospital system; using data available from different hospitals over varying periods, the death-rate in London hospitals averaged 41·72 per cent, in hospitals in large provincial towns 42·1 per cent, and in rural towns 44·92 per cent.[94]

The study of the operations performed at the General Infirmary at Leeds affords a breakdown of the different types of hernia treated between December 1852 and May 1867. A total of 111 operations are recorded – 'Of the 53 cases of inguinal, 34 recovered, 17 died; of the 54 cases of femoral, 37 recovered, 17 died; of the 4 cases of umbilical, 2 recovered, 2 died.'[95] The author believed:[96]

> that the greater proportion of successful femoral than of inguinal hernia operations is to be accounted for by the more acute and painful symptoms in strangulated femoral hernia inducing earlier attention and treatment than are given in the often long-standing inguinal form, in very many cases of which long delay and repeated violent attempts at reduction had induced gangrene of the gut before the patient was sent to the Infirmary. . . . The small number of umbilical hernia operations is well accounted for by the fact of so many cases in the end yielding to treatment; the great proportionate mortality in this form when the sac has to be opened, and the frequently chronic character of the symptoms, inducing every effort to be made to avoid operation.

Thus, yet again, the evidence suggests that even in this more common operation the repair of hernias was a comparatively rare event, and the success-rate varied from hospital to hospital and over time.

9   Hospital diseases

It cannot be surprising, if we look at the houses in which our forefathers lived in the sixteenth and seventeenth centuries, that their children in the eighteenth should be ignorant of all true principles of hospital construction or management; or that they should be impressed with any other idea than that which, in Miss Nightingale's words seemed to make it 'sufficient for all purposes of curing and healing, that the sick man and the doctor should merely be brought together, in any locality, or under any condition whatever.' But it is surprising to find that nearly a hundred years after Howard's vivid description of hospital misconstruction and management, and many years after the burning words of Florence Nightingale, that in a great hospital of six hundred beds we have been able to diminish the mortality only one per cent. from what it was in Howard's time. (Guy's Hospital mortality rate from 1780–90, 10·2 per cent.; 1850–60, 9·1 per cent.) If we go further back still, to the first five years of the existence of Guy's Hospital, we find the mortality 13·8 per cent. If we also bear in mind that then there were many zymotic diseases, now unknown, all of which were treated in the hospital, and almost only there, and that even of those which still remain to us cases are admitted to the hospital only by accident, and in a proportion which is infinitesimal (about 0·38 per cent.), the conclusion is inevitable that hospital hygiene has not advanced as it might and ought to have done.[1]

This lengthy comment on the salubrity of hospitals made by one of the foremost surgeons and gynaecologists in the last quarter of the nineteenth century is not as devastating as it might at first appear. The figures used to illustrate his case are overall mortality-rates and do not mention specifically deaths after surgical operations, which are peculiarly susceptible to 'hospital diseases', nor are figures included on mortality after the general introduction of antisepsis.

Pre-antisepsis

The earliest recognition of a hospital disease, probably typhus, was made by an army physician in the middle of the eighteenth century. The disease was caused, he thought, by 'a corruption of the air, pent up and deprived of its elastic parts by the respiration of a multitude; or more particularly vitiated with the perspirable matter, which, as it is the most volatile of the humours, is also the most putrescent'.[2] He considered that infection was derived from 'the poisonous effluvia of sores, mortifications, dysenteric and other putrid excrements'.[3]

A view published only a few years later found that:[4]

INFIRMARIES, or hospitals, in all countries, are for the most part unclean and infectious places, and tho' every precaution is taken to purify them, such as washing with vinegar, burning brimstone, gunpowder, or resinous substances, scouring the boards, and such like; yet a perfectly safe purification, in some cases can never be fully effected, unless after a great length of time; the seeds of infection once sown, continue in some instances, to spread contagious diseases, and to contaminate the house.

Similar points of view were taken up by two well-known physicians, Blizard and Aikin, at the end of the eighteenth century. The architect, wrote Aikin, wants to put the greatest number of patients into the least possible space, while the physician wants the largest amount of vacant space possible. However, the architect always wins, so:[5]

there is no doubt that it must become hurtful, when such a number, as from twenty to fifty persons, many of them afflicted with ulcers and other diseases which tend to aggravate the putrescency of the fluids, are constantly confined together in a room just large enough to hold their beds.

This attitude was reiterated by Blizard who wrote:[6]

Animal effluvia produce contagion. The pernicious impression of air, strongly impregnated therewith, is strikingly remarkable in compound fractures, and fractured sculls: but it is hurtful under all circumstances, however its effects may not be distinctly manifest, or the powers of the body may be superior to its influence. The circumstances of disease are generally polluting to the surrounding air.

These rather damning comments, based on a miasmatic view of contagion, appear to be strange in the context of hospital records, for in the minutes and annual reports of the hospitals little or no mention is made of hospital diseases as being a problem during the eighteenth century. They may, of course, not have wished to record the event, though in the nineteenth century cases are reported very fully. When hospitals were first established they were opened, naturally enough, in freshly cleaned and painted buildings, or even in purpose-built edifices; there were few accident cases admitted and the wards were not usually crowded, so the chances of the spread of infectious diseases were lessened. Thus, an historian of the Lincoln County Hospital wrote: 'I have the best authority for stating that in the earlier portion of its career, severe accidents usually did well, and that as to formidable operations it was quite the exception for them to prove fatal, or, indeed, for any serious complication to arise after their performance.'[7]

The Lincoln County Hospital was a country hospital and may have well had a different experience from other hospitals in the more densely populated areas, for in 1779 a surgeon wrote:[8]

By the exclusion of air many compound fractures, of late years, have been cured in a short time, and with little trouble. . . . It has been generally remarked that the cure of compound fractures does not succeed so well in the London hospitals as in the country, where the air is more pure and conducive to health.

This statement implies that the hospitals in the large towns were having trouble with infectious diseases in the second half of the eighteenth century, and this may have been true for some. The Liverpool Infirmary, for example, experienced difficulties from 1771 when new buildings were planned to give separate accommodation for patients suffering from venereal disease and to give more room in the building:[9]

to preserve the Lives and Health of the Apprentices, who have from the Commencement of the Charity, been so ill lodged in close Rooms and unwholesome Air that most of them have been endangered by the Hospital Fever; and one Youth indeed unhappily fell a sacrifice to this malignant Disease.

The problem was not cured by this extension and in 1780 galleries were built to improve the ventilation, but in 1782, despite the improvements, 'the bad consequences of a putrid air in retarding cases, particularly of ulcers, has not failed to manifest itself',[10] and the Infirmary was forced to restrict its admission:[11]

> Public Hospitals, particularly in a crowded metropolis, it is well known are not favourable to the cure of diseases; but as vice, poverty, and disease, will abound in such places, and many of the most wretched having no parish to which they can resort, hospitals become indispensable in such situations; and in country-towns, they serve as a receptacle for such poor as must undergo the more hazardous operations; and might be made the facts of general science, and become the means of diffusing useful knowledge amongst both sexes, throughout every part of the country.

This rationalization of the purpose of hospitals has a great deal of truth in it, for were conditions outside hospitals any better than those inside? This is doubtful from the contemporary descriptions of the life of the poor, particularly the urban poor, with the known unhygienic living conditions mainly resulting from overcrowding and the high density of population.[12]

> With all its faults and imperfections the 18th century hospital movement presents a noble effort to relieve suffering, an effort that by no means altogether failed in achievement. To many a poor sufferer the old, unreformed hospital with its warm bed, its pleasantly stuffy ward and its sufficiency of rough food must have been a harbour or refuge.

In the eighteenth century it needed the work of the naval physician, James Lind, and his associates to stress the importance of fresh air and cleanliness. Gradually the principles of reform spread through the hospitals; testers were removed, floors were scrubbed, cotton garments for patients and bed-linen were provided, cesspools and privies were investigated and improved, and the wooden beds were replaced by iron ones which did not harbour vermin.

The principal authority on the condition of hospitals at the end of the eighteenth century was John Howard, a philanthropic Quaker, who after a compaign for the reform of prisons, undertook a further challenge in attempting to improve the conditions in hospitals. His reports on the hospitals in England and Scotland showed great variations in the standards prevailing, showing that the process of change was slow and uneven.[13]

The overall impression given by the London hospitals with regard

to cleanliness was summarized by Howard in a rather caustic manner:
'White-washing the wards is seldom or never practised; and injurious
prejudices against washing floors, and admitting fresh air, are
suffered to operate.'[14] He, of course, was making a case for improvement, though, in fact, his reports do not fully support his
criticisms. However, the conditions in the London hospitals appear
to have been worse than those in the provincial hospitals. At
St Bartholomew's the wards were described as being 'clean and not
offensive', but the 'bedsteads are wood, and their testers, though
lofty, are a harbour for dust and lumber'.[15] Again, at St Thomas's
the wards were 'fresh and clean' except for three foul wards which
were 'very offensive and had not a window open'.[16] The old wards at
Guy's Hospital had wooden beds 'infested with bugs', but the new
wards had iron beds and water closets which were 'not in the least
offensive'.[17] St George's and the Westminster Hospital needed their
walls white-washing and the floors had been sanded instead of
scrubbed with water. Howard concluded his review of the London
hospitals with this statement:[18]

> I am fully persuaded that very much depends on the patients
> lying on fresh and clean beds. In many hospitals the beds are
> old, and crowded against the walls, so that there is no
> circulation of air round them; and, by a succession of patients
> with various disorders, must be very offensive. If the annual
> sum paid in several hospitals for the destruction of bugs, were
> expended in airing, beating and brushing the beds, the end,
> perhaps, would be much better answered. For in the country
> where the air is fresh, and freely admitted into lodging-rooms,
> there are few or no bugs.

The provincial hospitals, though not completely free from criticism, were subject to far less adverse comment. Presumably, this
was because of the smaller scale of operation of the hospitals in
country areas which also did not have the problems of overcrowding
which were to beset them in the nineteenth century. The Norfolk
and Norwich Hospital was described as being 'perfectly neat and
clean: the beds not crowded: the wards quiet and fresh'.[19] The
County Infirmaries at Leicester and Worcester were described as
'very close'[20] and 'offensive'[21] respectively. At Bath the Infirmary
was:[22]

> Cleaner and fresher than at my visit last year: several windows
> open; but many of the upper sashes do not let down, nor do

H

any of those in the passages or stair cases; which is the more necessary in such close and confined places as the site of this infirmary.

The Leeds Infirmary was described as 'one of the best hospitals in the kingdom . . . there is great attention to cleanliness. . . . There are no fixed testers: no bugs in the beds. Many are here cured of compound fractures, who would lose their limbs in the unventilated and offensive wards of some other hospitals.'[23]

The picture given by John Howard is thus a mixed one, not wholly good or wholly bad. It is evident that the hospitals, both in London and the provinces, did take account of the criticisms put forward by Howard. The London Hospital in Whitechapel Road took note and Howard remarked that 'By a letter lately received, I am informed that the committee are exerting themselves, and making several improvements in this hospital'.[24] He had criticized the practice of not separating the medical and surgical cases, though this was not peculiar to this hospital, and by an order made on 12 October 1790, the medical cases were separated: 'Agreed that two wards be set apart for the Physician's patients'. The Radcliffe Infirmary at Oxford came in for strong criticism for 'closeness and offensiveness' and Howard thought that 'The dry rubbing of the floors . . . is almost as bad as hiding the dirt with sand'.[25] One of the physicians to the Infirmary, in an open letter, defended the arrangements prevailing in the institution and attempted to counter each of Howard's criticisms. He concluded by stating:[26]

> To all these arguments let me add, that the house has been remarkably free from contagious fevers. I never remember one, which could be strictly laid to have originated here. They have sometimes been introduced by patients, inadvertently received, who had been brought from some place of confinement or some parish workhouse: but even in these cases, they have seldom spread, of which I could produce some very remarkable instances. This fact amounts to a demonstration, that the wards are not replete with noxious vapours, or an air favourable to the propagation of putrid fevers.

However, in 1790 plans were put forward for improvements to the ventilation of the building. When John Howard visited the Edinburgh Royal Infirmary he was informed that 'two or three years ago, a putrid fever prevailed in it; but that white-washing the walls had eradicated the infection, and that this salutary practice had been continued ever since'.[27]

The Manchester Infirmary, under the influence of John Aikin, its foremost physician, appears to have taken the cleanliness of its patients and of the institution very seriously from an early date, for in 1771 the following orders were given:[28]

1. That every patient has clean sheets upon their first admission.
2. That they have clean sheets at least once in three weeks.
3. That two patients be not suffered to be in the same bed except that there is no spare bed in the house.

Despite these measures, it was found necessary to discharge a number of the patients in 1788 as a slight fever had broken out in the house:[29]

A lengthy report from the Medical Officers followed, touching this prevailing unhealthiness, and an order was made to the effect: 1st – That proper openings for the admission of air were needed; 2nd – That the ceilings should be raised; 3rd – That iron beds should replace wooden ones; 4th – That the floors should be washed with soap and water, and no sand allowed to remain on them, also that doors and windows should be varnished; 5th – That five more Nurses should be engaged; 6th – That the wings of the Infirmary should be raised, and other additions for accommodating more patients, together with a diminution in the number of beds.

These recommendations would suggest that there had been an outbreak of one of the 'hospital diseases'. Certainly the overcrowding, poor ventilation and inadequate drainage would have contributed to this result.

Though the Newcastle Infirmary had forbidden the admission of infectious cases in 1774, it is evident that by the end of the eighteenth century the institution was experiencing the horrors of outbreaks of 'hospital diseases'. A contemporary description of the Infirmary stated that:[30]

The bedsteads are of wood, and badly situated, being placed with their sides against the wall. Two of the wards are too large, and all of them too much crowded. From a combination of circumstances of this nature, notwithstanding the favourable situation, the air of the Infirmary, in the morning, particularly, is impure.

Comparisons are made with other hospitals in Great Britain. Thus, at the General Infirmary at Leeds:[31]

> As great attention is paid to cleanliness and ventilation in every part of the house, and to the perfect repair of the water closets, the air of the Infirmary is not in general much less pure and healthy than in private homes. . . . It is a rule to change from one ward to another every two months.

Clark thought that the infirmaries at Manchester and Liverpool were 'well-regulated' as 'they have adopted the method of dividing the Medical from the Surgical patients; and by means of wards of different sizes, they are enabled to separate those cases which are offensive from the other patients'.[32] As he wished to illustrate in a vivid form the worst aspects of the Newcastle Infirmary the analysis was continued by examining the:[33]

> proportion of deaths, in compound fractures, fractures of the skull, and after amputation [which mark] more strongly the utility of ventilation, the advantages of different-sized wards, and the pernicious effects of vitiated air.
>   In the improved Infirmary at Northampton, the proportion of deaths after amputation, and from compound fractures, does not amount to one in 20; and in fractures of the skull, not more than one in 8.

At the General Infirmary at Leeds:[34]

> From March 1799, to May 1801, 30 amputations have been performed, with the loss of one patient only. Two or three patients with fractures are received into the house weekly; seldom more than 8 compound fractures in a year: But not one has died of fractures of any kind during the last 12 months.

> In the Infirmary at Glasgow, the proportion of deaths appears to be about one in 20, from fractures; and after amputations, one in 12.

> In the large hospitals in the metropolis, where numbers are crowded together, and where it will almost be impossible, with every contrivance, to preserve the air pure and untainted, the success of amputation, of the treatment of compound fractures, or fractures of the skull, is much less than in the modern improved hospitals, plainly evincing that purity of air is essential

to the fortunate event of operations, and that even increased skill and knowledge of the profession will not counterbalance the want of it.

In the Newcastle Infirmary, during the last two years, 59 cases of simple and compound fractures have been admitted, 9 of who died, being in the proportion nearly of one in 6; and in fractures of the skull, 6 have been admitted, and 5 have died. And although it must be observed, that those who died of compound fractures, and fractures of the skull, were cases of the worst kind; yet more of them might probably have recovered in smaller and better ventilated wards.

He concluded: 'Such is the difference in the success of the practice between old and improved Infirmaries, that no one can for a moment hesitate in ascribing it to cleanliness, ventilation, and proper accommodation'.[35]

The case at the Edinburgh Royal Infirmary towards the end of the eighteenth century is a little confused. One of the surgeons, on the pessimistic side, wrote that:[36]

Our surgical patients are exposed to infections from the Medical Wards, and especially to a disease, the Hospital sore, which seizes all those who have even the smallest incisions practised upon them: it infects all the ulcers, changes the slightest sores into gangrenes; and this disease, which is frequent in exact proportion to the size of an Hospital, is so peculiar, that it is named Hospital-gangrene. It is like a plague; it rages twice a year in such a degree, that the nurses even are infected; the lightest scratch in their fingers turns out a most formidable sore, and at certain seasons no operation can be safely performed.

However, this statement was denied by Mr Russell, Senior Surgeon to the Royal Infirmary, who wrote 'that a very small number of the patients under my care have suffered from the complaint; and that the cases have in general been slight, and of little consequence. It has never appeared under a contagious form, by attacking a number of patients at a time'.[37] In defence of the Royal Infirmary Dr Gregory, the physician, wrote:[38]

that sometimes, from neglect of due ventilation and cleanliness in the Surgeons Wards, the patients in them suffered severely;

a slight wound or ulcer in many cases degenerating into a bad
spreading sore of great extent, scarce to be healed, sometimes
running to gangrene, and attended with fever, and ultimately
proving fatal. I understood likewise, that, in many instances,
operations seemingly well performed, had soon proved fatal,
from the same causes: instead of good suppuration and healing,
bad spreading ulceration, and gangrene, and fever,
supervening upon them. I understood even that such bad
condition of wounds or ulcers had sometimes spread in the
Surgeons Wards of this Hospital, as in other hospitals,
seemingly by contagion. I knew that this did not happen always,
or even generally in this Hospital.

Gregory continued by examining the types of cases admitted to the
Edinburgh Royal Infirmary:[39]

Some patients are occasionally admitted into the common
medical and clinical wards, with simple, or scrofulous, or
syphilitic, or cancerous ulcers; and hundreds of patients in
these wards, every year, undergo slight incisions or wounds, by
bleeding, either with the lancet or with leeches, or by cupping
and scarifying, by opening imposthumes, by puncturing, or by
tapping for dropsies of different kinds; and worse than all,
undergo ample excoriation, by blisters, without getting
hospital-gangrene, or anything like it; nay such excoriations and
small incisions, as by bleeding with the lancet or leeches, are
often performed on patients actually labouring under the
infectious fever, without inducing any hospital-gangrene.

Thus, it would appear that the end of the eighteenth century, though
hospital-gangrene was occurring at the Edinburgh Royal Infirmary,
it did not manifest itself in an epidemic form. This may well have
been the case for the other voluntary hospitals at the time. Certainly,
the lack of evidence and of contemporary literature would suggest
this point of view.

The turn into the nineteenth century saw a dramatic change in the
incidence of 'hospital diseases':

As might have been anticipated, coincidently with the growth
of the population there came an increased strain upon the
Hospital resources, and then, by degrees, special defects in the
construction of the Hospital, of small consequence when the
inmates were few, assumed great importance when these

became numerous. Such defects rendered it impossible to preserve a sufficient degree of purity in the air of the wards, or to prevent its contamination by emanations from cesspools. The water-supply also became polluted. Hence arose outbreaks of pyaemia, erysipelas, sloughing of wounds, and intractable diarrhoea, maladies which were evidently due to faults in the Hospital itself, as they were not coincident with epidemics of similar affections outside its walls.[40]

These disasters naturally excited very great anxiety in the minds of the Governors, and various attempts were, from time to time, made by them to improve the sanitary condition of the Institution.[41]

These comments on the experience of the Lincoln County Hospital are applicable to virtually every hospital in the United Kingdom during the nineteenth century until the general introduction and adoption of Listerian antiseptic techniques in the last quarter of the century. Examination of the records of the voluntary hospitals and of the contemporary literature shows that one after the other the hospitals fell to the dreaded 'hospital disease'.

It spread to the smallest hospital. In 1803 the Salisbury General Infirmary suffered, for in that year the Weekly Board congratulated themselves on new arrangements in the wards enabling them 'to remove some inconveniences experienced by patients with fractured limbs'.[42]

An outbreak of erysipelas during the two years 1821 and 1822 at the Edinburgh Royal Infirmary is of interest as the measures used to counteract the infection have been well documented. An Extraordinary Meeting was convened on 30 July 1821 when the surgeons requested that 'those Patients at present affected with Erysipelas [be] removed to some other Wards, both surgical and Medical Patients being affected'.[43] The disease appeared again in January 1822 when:[44]

the Managers directed that the Sailors' Ward shall be opened, and that the Surgeons shall at the same time be requested to endeavour to prevent their Wards from being so crowded as they are at present, and to keep in view that the Sailors' Ward is to be used exclusively for Patients attacked with the Erysipelas.

It had disappeared by July 1822, but again appeared in September of that year. There was a proposal that no further patients should be admitted, but the Medical Officers did not feel that this was the best policy, though they admitted that 'we are acquainted with no means to prevent its recurrence besides ventilation and cleanliness particularly of the bedding to which too much attention cannot be paid'.[45]

A complete re-building programme was undertaken in the early years of the 1820s at the General Infirmary at Leeds, and it was found that as a result the number of cases of hospital-gangrene was lessened because of the increased space and ventilation available for the patients.[46] For the year 1822 at the Glasgow Royal Infirmary:[47]

The cases which supervened upon other diseases and which proved fatal, amount to 13, 1 in 14·53. . . . From this it will appear that Erysipelas is far from being so mortal a distemper as some others, such as dropsy or consumption. The whole mortality by Erysipelas being 1 in 9·04 deaths occurring in the course of a year.

Despite this statement, it is interesting to note that the number of cases of erysipelas increases year by year from the opening of the Glasgow Royal Infirmary, there being 9 in 1795 and in 1822 there were 59 cases.[48]

The General Infirmary at Sheffield fell victim to sepsis in 1825 when:[49]

the house fever appeared in a very dangerous form, so that the patients called it the 'black fever'. Richard, the porter, died of it; and Mr Atkinson, the apprentice, suffered from it very severely. It was found necessary to empty the house nearly, and to whitewash and cleanse it throughout. Notwithstanding all these means of improving the state of the wards, sloughing sores, after operations, did not cease to occur during that and subsequent years. Sometimes, indeed, it was found impossible to heal these sores and hence the sufferers were obliged to be dismissed uncured, to the discredit of the institution. It is particularly in regard to these sloughing cases that the foul state of the house is evinced, as the following facts will very abundantly show:—During the last four months of 1825, the year in which the thorough cleansing was had recourse to, and during 1826 and part of 1827, out of fourteen persons that suffered amputation of the limbs by two of the surgeons, no less than the extraordinary number of six died. Extraordinary, be it said, for, we believe, it is pretty well known, that under favourable circumstances, the ordinary mortality, in such cases, is not more than ONE in TWENTY or THIRTY. And, at this moment [1833], the average mortality, we are informed, continues about ONE in THREE or FOUR!! and for the last four years at least, there has not been a single week without a case of sloughing in the house! . . . In the spring of the present year [1833] the defective state of the ventilation became, once more, very apparant. Sloughing sores and erysipelas prevailed, and one of the house apprentices very nearly fell a victim to the latter. Mr. Staniforth (the surgeon) and his colleagues made strong complaints in person at the Weekly Board; for they found themselves placed in this very awkward predicament: they had patients requiring the performance of operation, which however, they actually dared not undertake for fear of the consequences.

On 3 May 1833 it was ordered that no medical cases were to be admitted as in-patients from that date. Thus, the Sheffield General Infirmary was severely attacked by the 'hospital diseases', and the statement of the surgeons of the infirmary illustrates in a vivid form the lack of knowledge about the causes of sepsis and the resultant inability to deal with the situation, except for the traditional cleansing and white-washing.

A report was made by the authorities at the Salisbury General Infirmary on its defective state in 1831:[50]

The Drains were found to be so badly constructed, as not to admit of improvement; consequently, new ones have been made. The Closets also, and the mode of ventilation, have been so improved that the Auditors trust that they will be found fully to answer the purposes intended, and leave no room for complaint in future.

However, a further outbreak of erysipelas occurred only two years later in 1833 and the medical staff made a number of recommendations which were put into effect. As a result of these measures the hospital was free of infection within three months.[51]

In 1834 at the Birmingham General Hospital it was found that 'In consequence of the prevalence of Erysipelas amongst the patients during part of the past years, it has been thought desirable to cause the Hospital to undergo a thorough purification. This is completed, and the house is now quite free from infectious complaints.'[52]

A lecturer at the Leeds School of Medicine, writing in 1841 on hospital diseases, stated that there was:[53]

> hardly a large hospital in which the disease [erysipelas] has not formerly prevailed to such an extent as in many cases, to render the closing of the whole or part of the wards requisite: as St. Thomas's and St. George's Hospital in London; the Leeds Infirmary, and the Birmingham Hospital, in the country; the Montrose and Edinburgh Infirmaries, in Scotland.

Of hospital-gangrene, he considered that:[54]

> The greater attention now paid to hygienic considerations, has so diminished the appearance of hospital gangrene, that it but rarely comes under the notice of the mere civilian, at least in a severe form, or as an epidemic; and in these piping times of peace is not very often presented to the military surgeon.

The comment that improved ventilation and cleanliness had solved all the problems was, unfortunately, far from the truth of the situation, particularly after the introduction of anaesthesia in 1846 when the incidence of hospital disease increased with the rise in the amount and complexity of surgical operations performed.

It is worth while examining the causes of death after surgical operations in the period prior to the introduction of anaesthesia. At Guy's Hospital between 19 May 1827 and 19 May 1842 there were 153 deaths in cases of patients who 'had undergone severe operations, or suffered from extensive accidental injuries'.[55] 134 died of 'inflammation of secreting surfaces or internal organs (excluding the kidneys, liver and spleen)', while only 19 died 'from other causes, such as tetanus, sloughing, haemorrhage, suppuration, gangrene, erysipelas, diarrhoea, and the total deficiency of reparative action in the wound'.[56] The comment was made that 'the air and ventilation are tolerably good' and that 'secondary fever and the worst forms of erysipelas are not prevalent in the surgical wards'.[57] As the presence of hospital diseases was not noticed in the wards it was concluded that 'the chances of death after operation etc. appear to depend almost entirely upon the previous state of each patient's constitution'.[58]

A survey conducted again at Guy's Hospital in 1859, i.e. after the general use of anaesthetic techniques was widespread, found that in 300 cases of amputation pyaemia (another form of sepsis) was 'the cause of death in 42 per cent. of all fatal cases of amputation and in

10 per cent. of all amputations'.[59] It was the cause of death 'in 70 per cent. of all fatal amputations of expediency; in 43 per cent. of all fatal pathological amputations; in 25 per cent. of all fatal secondary amputations; and that in amputations of expediency it is the most frequent cause, in secondary amputations the least'.[60]

This striking increase in the incidence of one of the forms of hospital disease as a cause of death was reflected in the experience of hospitals throughout the country, particularly during the third quarter of the nineteenth century. Two examples will illustrate the point; one a hospital in a large provincial town, the Birmingham General Hospital; and one a hospital in a small county town, the York County Hospital.

The General Hospital in Birmingham was continually suffering from the problems attendant upon overcrowding and matters came to a head in 1859 with a report from a Special Medical Board:[61]

In the opinion of this Board, the number of beds now occupied by patients is too great in several of the wards of the Hospital, and for a long period the Institution has been overcrowded, not only by the number of beds already in use, but also by extra beds placed on the floor for the reception of the numerous applicants for medical or surgical relief. . . . The inevitable results of this overcrowding have manifested themselves in various ways; as evidenced by the lengthened period occupied in the process of cure, and in many instances by the development, from time to time of diseases of a low type.

Large extensions were recommended, and a new wing was built. However, the problem persisted and in December 1862 a report was made on 'the bad sanitary state of the Hospital, as manifested by the unhealthy appearance of wounds, etc., and the slow recovery of patients suffering from them'. The Report recommended the rejection of all In-Patients recommended by Subscribers, excepting those whose cases were very urgent.[62] This was put into effect, but the improvement in the state of the building was temporary for in 1864 a further report was published – 'The state of the Hospital, as regards accommodation for its household, has still been sadly defective, consequently many of them suffered from sickness, and for one month an average of five persons were prevented from attending to their duties from illness contracted within the walls of the Hospital'.[63] The number of beds was cut further and extensions were constructed and improvements made, including 'the addition of four Wards for infectious cases and burns'.[64] In 1874 a new drainage system was installed and in the following year the Medical Committee proudly reported 'that the Hospital has been very free from epidemic disease during the past year. . . . The few attacks of erysipelas which have occurred in the Hospital, have taken place in those peculiar kinds of injury which are especially prone to take on such action, even under favourable circumstances.'[65]

At the York County Hospital evidence was submitted to the Governors to consider the necessity for a new building in 1846. During the previous winter there had been great pressure on the resources of the hospital and it was reported that:[66]

> Surgical cases were obliged to be injuriously intruded into the
> medical wards; [and] that the impossibility of allotting separate
> accommodation to cases of painful, or fetid disease, was a
> source of great disturbance and annoyance to the other patients,
> and that within a few weeks, the necessity, owing to the want of
> separate wards, for removing a patient whose wounds were in a
> state of gangrene, to the operation room, on account of the
> offensiveness of their smell, had caused the postponement of an
> operation which ought, had it been practicable, to have been
> sooner performed.

There had already been a report from a special committee in 1840 on the state of the building which recommended a larger establishment.[67] A further report was issued in 1852 on warming and ventilation, in which it was noted that 'In the Visitors' Book for the last six months are three entries in which notice is taken of a disagreeable smell, they are each specifically stated as occurring in the Surgeon's Ward, and in one traced to the bed-side of a patient suffering under gangrenous ulcer'.[68] Six years later 'it was stated by the Medical Officers that Erysipelas of a highly contagious kind exists in the Hospital, so that it has been found necessary to close the male surgical ward and to send the most important surgical cases out of the Hospital'.[69] In the middle of 1859 erysipelas was present again and it was thought desirable to close the hospital 'for a period of not less than two months, and, in the meantime, be thoroughly white washed and cleaned'.[70] This was put into effect in October of that year.[71] It was in the same year that the artificial system of ventilation used in the hospital was discontinued; 'windows which had been formerly kept closed were henceforward habitually opened; open fire-places, of which there had been none, were provided . . . and since then the place has continued perfectly healthy'.[72]

These seemingly bad conditions in hospitals, particularly after the introduction of anaesthesia, led to a flood of literature on the salubrity and the suitability of the hospitals to perform their functions properly. In 1866 two extensive articles were published in the *British and Foreign Medico-Chirurgical Review*, reviewing the new books and articles on the construction of hospitals, as well as their siting and ventilation. Ten individual works were considered;[73] they were the most influential works of the period and illustrate the concern felt about the state of hospitals at this time.

The studies give rise to distinctions between healthy and unhealthy hospitals: 'A hospital which does not by any fault of its own aggravate ever so little the recovery of persons who are properly its inmates' can be described as healthy, while in another hospital:[74]

by means of some faults of its own disease cannot be treated as successfully as in the other hospital; and the fault of its own through which an 'unhealthy' hospital fails to attain the best results for its medical and surgical treatment, is of two kinds – either it is inherent, as of site and construction; or else it is a fault of keeping, as dirtiness, or overcrowding, or neglect of ventilation.

Florence Nightingale, having earlier campaigned for the proper training of nurses, turned her attention in the early 1860s to the state of hospitals. Her influential book[75] provoked the nation's conscience, her impassioned plea for radical change was extremely effective in that a government inquiry[76] was instituted in the same year:[77]

If the recovery of the sick simply is to be the object of hospitals, they will not be built among dense, unhealthy population. . . . Land in towns is too expensive for hospitals to be so built as to secure the conditions of ventilation and of light, and of spreading the inmates over a large surface-area – conditions now known to be essential to speedy recovery – instead of piling them up three or four stories high, in regions contaminated with coal-smoke and nuisances.

Her views were accepted by many of the foremost authorities,[78] but she continued her argument and went on to advocate the pavilion type of construction:[79]

The essential feature of the pavilion construction is that of breaking up hospitals of any size into a number of separate detached parts, having a common administration, but nothing else in common. And the object sought is that the atmosphere of no one pavilion or ward should diffuse itself to any other pavilion or ward, but should escape into the open air as speedily as possible, whilst its place is supplied by the purest obtainable air from the outside.

However, Miss Nightingale was not supported by the report of J. S. Bristowe and T. Holmes, either in the siting of hospitals or in their planning. Of the siting of hospitals, they made the following comment:[80]

That there might be some variation in the mortality may or may not be probable, but that the prevalence of hospital disease would be much decreased, that operations on given cases would be much abridged, we do, judging from the evidence before us of the state of things in hospitals variously circumstanced as far as situation goes, disbelieve.

This was in spite of the evidence taken from a report to the Governors of St George's Hospital that even in this hospital:[81]

unrivalled for its situation in this or any other city, in a ward well placed for air and ventilation, one of the scourges of surgical disease, phagadaena [sloughing sores and wounds], has been exceedingly prevalent during the past season. To be enabled to send away patients for the further treatment they may require when such a disease makes its appearance would certainly result in the saving of many lives.

On the question of the planning of hospitals Bristowe and Holmes were rather negative, but they admitted that:[82]

where the wards are small and close, and the corridors are long, narrow, irregular in direction or shape, and ill ventilated, we believe it to be true that they do oppose a very serious obstacle to the free ventilation of the wards, and have a direct tendency to the production of hospital diseases, and these defects of construction may, we believe, be traced to have had such influence in hospitals like those of Leeds, Lincoln, Manchester, &c.

The principal reasons given by the two authors for not approving of the pavilion system of hospital-building were 'the distance of parts of the hospital from each other', and 'the costliness of the construction'.[83] Thus, although Bristowe and Holmes found great failings in the older hospitals they did not feel that the pavilion system was feasible.

This dispute on the rights and wrongs of various types of hospital construction and siting was based on a series of conflicting statistics collected by a number of authorities. Bristowe and Holmes collected figures on the incidence of 'hospital diseases' which were present at the time that the authors visited the hospitals. Before examining the figures it should be noted that these are given for one day only in each hospital, i.e. the day that they were visited, and that the figures, therefore, may not accurately reflect the true running of the hospital as the prevalence of infection was susceptible to fluctuation. The conclusions reached were that:[84]

> out of every 100 surgical patients in the metropolitan hospitals 1·9, out of every 100 in the provincial hospitals 1·7, and out of every 100 in rural hospitals ·7, suffering from erysipelas, phagadaena, or pyaemia contracted in hospital.

> The statistics prove little, still that little is in favour of the opinion we have expressed, to the effect that the presence of these affections is dependent less on the kind and position of a hospital than it is on the severity and number of cases likely to be affected by them.

> At first sight it may appear that the rural hospitals have a decided advantage, but it must not be forgotten that phagadaena and diffused inflammation have . . . been unusually prevalent during the period which our inquiry embraced, among patients applying for relief at London Hospitals.

In an attempt to be more specific an analysis was made of deaths from pyaemia in both London and rural hospitals. Pyaemia was chosen as:[85]

> hospital erysipelas and phagadaena are so rarely fatal, that no result whatever would have been yielded even by the most careful analysis we might have made in regard to them; and that even as respects pyaemia the results are far from

trustworthy, especially in the cases of country hospitals where post-mortem inquiries into the causes of death are rarely instituted.

The figures were taken principally for the year 1862 and the authors found, surprisingly, that 3·4 per cent of total deaths in rural hospitals were caused by pyaemia, while only 1·7 per cent of total deaths in London hospitals were from this cause. The most important fact to emerge from their study was that 'pyaemia is, both in town and country, actually an infrequent cause of death when compared with all other causes of death, and with the total number of patients admitted for treatment',[86] even when an allowance was made for any inaccuracy in the records. For Guy's Hospital (two years), St Thomas's (two years), and St George's, whose records were considered to be accurate, the authors found that 21 deaths from pyaemia had occurred out of a total of 1,696 patients who died among the 18,097 who had been admitted for treatment. 'The deaths from pyaemia formed, therefore, 1·23 per cent of the total number of deaths, and the death-rate due to pyaemia was 0·115 per cent.'[87]

These conclusions were at variance with the sensational outburst of Florence Nightingale and other authorities. The main protagonist was Sir James Young Simpson who, in a series of articles, attempted to prove that amputations performed in country practices were safer than those performed in large and metropolitan hospitals. By an odd assorted collection of statistics he found that out of 2,098 amputations performed in country practice only 226 patients died. The excess of deaths in hospital practice, he considered, pleaded 'eloquently and clamantly for a revision and reform of our existing hospital system'.[88] He thought that 'our system of huge and colossal hospital edifices . . . counteracts and cancels all the advances and improvements which modern surgical and medical science has evoked'.[89] The statistics used by Sir James Young Simpson to support his case were treated with some suspicion on their publication and many authorities came forward to furnish figures from their own hospitals.[90] Thus, for example, at the General Infirmary at Leeds, in the six months from 1 May 1865 to 31 October 1865 there were 21 fatalities out of 100 recorded operations; while from 1 October 1868 to 31 March 1869 out of 140 operations there were only 6 deaths recorded.[91] The comment on these figures was that:[92]

seeing the number of patients in the hospital was the same in each period, there surely must have been some potent unseen cause influencing the result; mere 'hospitalism' will not account for it. In the last period, when there was the largest number of operations and the greatest crowding the fatality was the least. Moreover, the last months of the hospital, which had been above a hundred years in use, were far more healthy than many periods which had occurred during its long occupation.

Though the figures were quite favourable as regards the total number of deaths from 'hospital diseases', the fact remains that many of the hospital authorities were concerned about the hygiene and ventilation of their institutions.[93]

As an illustration, the authorities at the Manchester Royal Infirmary made a considerable number of changes to the internal arrangements of the hospital, particularly in the 1860s after a report from a medical sub-committee in 1861:[94]

Notwithstanding these great changes the surgical wards were 'unhealthy' during five months of 1863, and two months of 1864; and in the autumn of 1865, 'several cases of sloughing were reported', apparently a slighter form of hospital gangrene, and the beginning of an outbreak of that disease which affected the wards in the two following years. In 1866, there were noted in the surgical wards 21 cases of pyaemia, of which 13 were fatal; also, cases of 'sloughing' and 'phagedaena' (in other words, I take it, hospital gangrene) in June, September, and November, 'several cases' in each of the two latter months. Four of the deaths from pyaemia happened in December, when the surgical wards were stated to have been 'very unhealthy'. The next year, 1867, was one of the unhealthiest in the annals of the Infirmary. During five months of the year, January, February, March, May, and June, 'hospital gangrene' was present in the surgical wards, part of the time with pyaemia and erysipelas; and of pyaemia, 15 cases were recorded, 10 fatal, distributed throughout the several months of the year, except June and October. In 1868, eight cases of 'sloughing' and one of 'hospital gangrene' (July) were recorded in the surgical wards; also three fatal cases of pyaemia and two cases of erysipelas. After this year 'hospital gangrene' seems to have disappeared from the wards.

Following these outbreaks partitions were removed and fever and convalescent hospitals were opened:[95]

I

but in 1874 another period of ward unhealthiness commenced, hardly, if at all, less serious in its character than previously recorded periods of unhealthiness. Towards the close of 1874 the surgical wards having been more or less 'unhealthy' since June of that year, but in what particular way is not stated, erysipelas became common in them. This malady continued prevalent in these wards during 1875, and to the time of this inquiry in June 1876, and it appeared also to some extent in the medical wards, and in the ward especially reserved for diseases of women, under the obstetric physician. According to the Infirmary register, three cases of pyaemia, one of septicaemia, and 11 cases of erysipelas, originated in the surgical wards, in 1874; two cases of pyaemia, three of septicaemia, and 36 cases of erysipelas, in 1875; and one case of pyaemia, one of septicaemia, and 29 cases of erysipelas from 1st January to the 12th June inclusive of the present year (1876).

With a long history of unhealthiness the Lincoln County Hospital again came under the influence of 'hospital diseases' in 1860:[96]

> The troublesome and expensive process of stoving the wards, from which much apparent benefit had previously been derived, was again resorted to, but, on this occasion, without success. The object of this process was so thoroughly to heat the wards, and the beds and bedding they contained, as effectually to destroy any disease germs they might be supposed to harbour. . . . For three or four days the temperature was maintained at 180° or higher, after which the windows were thrown open for a short time, and the ward was then considered fit to be reoccupied.

Despite this treatment, the hospital had to be evacuated and temporary accommodation taken for the more urgent cases. Dr J. S. Bristowe was engaged to report on the hospital, in which he concluded that it 'is not, and cannot be brought up to the standard of modern requirements'.[97] A decision to rebuild was taken in January 1874 and the new building was opened in October 1878.

This last example of a hospital suffering under the ravages of 'hospital diseases', which was typical of many at the time, added fuel to the flames in the arguments of John Erichsen of University College Hospital who sensationalized the whole topic of 'hospitalism'. In addition to the evidence presented on the Lincoln County

Hospital given by T. Sympson, John Erichsen found that in 80 consecutive cases of amputation (excluding all partial amputations of hand and foot) performed at University College Hospital between 1 July 1870 and 1 December 1873, 'there were 3 deaths from shock (all primary), and 10 from pyaemia and erysipelas leaving only 8 deaths to be accounted for by exhaustion and the other minor and more varied causes'.[98] He went on to examine other statistical evidence, and as a result of his researches he concluded that hospital influences 'give rise to the septic diseases that are so fatal, pyaemia alone being the cause of death in more than one-third of the fatal cases; and, if this could be removed, we should be able to lessen our mortality proportionately'.[99] However, it should be noted that these alarming figures could easily be misconstrued as they were taken out of context. The number of deaths and causes of death must be considered in relation to the total number of patients admitted to a hospital, to the number of surgical operations performed (which was a small percentage of the total number of cases treated); and the number of surgical deaths must be related to the total number of deaths.

Antisepsis

It would seem extraordinary that the paper of Erichsen should be published in 1874, and others of a similar nature in the 1880s,[100] when the work of Pasteur on bacteria had been established, and Joseph Lister had investigated the possibility of finding an agent which would prevent infection from entering a wound, particularly a surgical wound, with the resultant discovery of an effective antiseptic in 1865. In his famous paper in the *Lancet*[101] Lister related that he was struck by the effectiveness of carbolic acid, which had been added to the sewage of Carlisle, in 'destroying the entozoa which usually infect cattle'[102] which fed on the pastures which had been irrigated with refuse material. His first attempt on a case of compound fracture of the leg in March 1865 at the Glasgow Royal Infirmary was unsuccessful because of 'improper management; but subsequent trials have more than realized my most sanguine anticipations'.[103] His use of carbolic acid, in the early stages, was to swab the wound, thereby killing the germs in the wound and erecting a barrier against the entry of further bacteria. This method used by Lister was dependent on the antiseptic drug, carbolic acid, and his method was therefore antisepsis. His principle, however, was to erect a barrier against bacteria entering the wound, therefore his principle was one of asepsis. Of the first eleven patients on which he reported in this article only one died, though not from sepsis, although two were attacked by a 'hospital disease' but subsequently recovered.

In April 1867 Joseph Lister started to use antisepsis in his performance of surgical operations at the Glasgow Royal Infirmary and the figures on its success are quite startling. In the years 1864 to 1866 Lister operated on 35 cases for amputation, of which 16 were fatal; while from 1867 to 1869, using antiseptic techniques, of 40 cases operated on only 6 died. Joseph Lister, commenting on these figures, wrote:[104]

> We have seen that a degree of salubrity equal to that of the best private houses has been attained in peculiarly unhealthy wards of a very large hospital, by simply enforcing strict attention to the antiseptic principle. And, considering the circumstances of those wards, it seems hardly too much to expect that the same beneficent change which has passed over them will take place in all surgical hospitals, when the principle shall be similarly recognised and acted on by the profession generally.

The method used by Lister was simple, but its success depended on the rigid application of every detail, and this lack of detail may have accounted for the relative disappointment of many surgeons about the antiseptic principle. A survey made by the *Lancet* in 1868–9 showed that every large London hospital and some of the provincial hospitals had taken up the technique, but with varying degrees of success. For example, a report from St George's Hospital in 1868 on forty cases of compound fractures, lacerated wounds, incised wounds (including surgical operations), abscesses, and burns and scalds concluded that no positive statement could be made 'but at any rate the treatment has not proved either painful or dangerous'.[105] Lister explained that 'whatever be the antiseptic means employed . . . use them so as to render impossible the existence of a living septic organism in the part concerned'.[106] This meant acceptance of the germ theory, which many refuted, and also on the complete adherence to the principle of antisepsis. Lister moved to Edinburgh in 1869 and reported on his experiences during the first nine months at the Royal Infirmary:[107]

I have as yet had no instance of pyaemia, although many
cases have been admitted in which it might, under ordinary
treatment, have been apprehended, such as compound
fractures, amputations in the lower limb, and extensive gouging
operations upon bone. Hospital gangrene also has been
entirely absent. Though several cases of ulcers of long
standing have been under treatment, there has never been any
appearance of greyness of the surface to indicate even the
mildest form of the disease.

Despite the evident success of antisepsis as demonstrated by Lister,
the method took a considerable number of years to be generally
adopted. There were two principal reasons for the slow spread of
Lister's work: first, Lister did not move to London (King's College
Hospital) until 1877; and second, there was great opposition to the
antiseptic method from some vociferous critics, including the
famous surgeon and gynaecologist Robert Lawson Tait. Although
Lawson Tait claimed equal success while not using antisepsis, in
fact, he did practise a form of asepsis by washing his instruments
and his hands before commencing an operation. The germ theory
was the main impediment to acceptance of the antiseptic principle,
and it was this that had to be acknowledged before Lister's work
could be implemented.

A fitting conclusion to this chapter can be taken from the work of
the surgeon Timothy Holmes who, writing in the mid-1870s, stated
that 'no doubt the popular impression of the frequency of pyaemia
in our hospitals is extremely exaggerated'.[108] He continued by
lamenting:[109]

the exaggerated importance (as I at last believe) the writings of
Miss Nightingale and other hospital authorities, who have
followed in her wake, have attributed to the details of hospital
construction, such as size, cubic space, arrangement of pavilions,
ventilation, &c., and the expectations they have held out that
by improvements effected in these details we might expect to
lessen very materially the death-rate of our operations.

His acceptance of the work of Joseph Lister was qualified, like
many surgeons, though this did not diminish his admiration of
Lister's achievement:[110]

It was a true surgical instinct that led Professor Lister to look
to the after-management of the case for the means of

diminishing, as far as might be, the mortality in an unselected series of amputations; and I think that we can trace a sensible diminution of mortality since 'the antiseptic method' has come into vogue. . . . Irrespective of any theories about the cause of putrefaction, or the influence on the progress of the case which is exercised by the putrefaction of the surfaces of a wound, no one doubts the great importance of scrupulous cleanliness, minute attention to all the details of dressing, and careful avoidance of any unnecessary meddling with the wound.

Thus, the experience of hospitals with regard to the infection of patients admitted in the eighteenth and nineteenth centuries can be divided roughly into three time-periods. First, the period prior to 1800 when any unhygienic conditions or practices were not of great importance as there was little overcrowding and very few operations were performed. The likelihood of sepsis was, therefore, extremely limited. Second, the period after 1800 to the late 1860s when the hospitals experienced great pressure on their limited resources with consequent overcrowding. In addition, after the general introduction of anaesthesia in the mid-1840s the numbers and scope of surgery increased and the conditions in hospitals became alarmingly bad for a small proportion of the patients, i.e., those undergoing surgical operations. However, hospitals could find that there would be no trouble from any of the 'hospital diseases' for a number of years and then suddenly they would have to experience the tragedy of a short period of great infection. Third, the period after Joseph Lister had demonstrated the antiseptic principle. Despite the opposition to Lister real progress was made, albeit slowly, in the management of surgical patients, both during and after the operation, and in the general conditions prevailing in hospitals.

Although antisepsis was superseded by the principle of asepsis, i.e. a completely germ-free environment so there is no need for antiseptic measures to be taken, the work of Joseph Lister proved to be a turning-point in the development of modern surgery. It was during the last quarter of the nineteenth century and the first quarter of the twentieth that great advances were made. These could only be undertaken without the fear of one of the 'hospital diseases' supervening.

10   Gateways to death?

Medical historians have tended to view the hospitals in the eighteenth and nineteenth centuries as being horrific institutions in which most of the patients died. This dismissal of the work of the voluntary hospitals has been stated in the strongest of terms:[1]

> Indeed, the chief indictment of hospital work at this period is not that it did no good, but that it positively did harm . . . The common cause of death was infectious disease; any patient admitted to hospital faced the risk of contracting a mortal infection . . . it was not until much later [than the eighteenth century] that hospital patients could be reasonably certain of dying from the disease with which they were admitted.

However, the evidence upon which this damning conclusion is based needs to be examined, particularly in the light of the facts which have been presented in previous chapters. The practice of St Bartholomew's Hospital of admitting cholera patients to the general wards in 1854 is used to support the view that hospitals did not appreciate the necessity of separating infectious and non-infectious cases. This is highly misleading, for the hospitals varied in their attitudes towards infectious disease and policies changed according to experience. 'Contemporary accounts of the unsatisfactory conditions in eighteenth century hospitals . . . in the writings of Percival, Howard, etc.'[2] are given as further evidence without any form of criticism. Although John Howard found that conditions in the London hospitals were not above reproach, his reports on the provincial hospitals he visited disclose a mixed picture of good and bad conditions.[3] There is, however, a footnote reference which suggests that conditions in London hospitals were worse than those in one Parisian hospital in 1788.[4] This is of great interest when in 1808 it was found that at the Hôtel Dieu in Paris mortality was one in five, while in no English hospital did the rate exceed one in eleven.[5] On the mortality after surgery, evidence is taken from a book, published in 1874,[6] by the senior surgeon at University College Hospital, John Erichsen.[7]

He showed that mortality following all form of amputation was between 35% and 50%, and following certain [unspecified] forms it was as high as 90%. Results of other types of operation were equally bad; Erichsen's observations were based upon the third quarter of the nineteenth century; there is no reason to suppose that earlier results were better.

The notion that these high rates of surgical mortality were preceded by even higher rates in the eighteenth century is highly misleading. Mortality after surgery in the early years of hospital practice was not high, and even the figures presented by John Erichsen were not representative of the voluntary hospitals in the third quarter of the nineteenth century.

Florence Nightingale, in a perfect example of the abuse of statistics, attempted to show that mortality in hospitals was disgracefully high and that improvements would have to be made. A reviewer of her book[8] wrote that 'It is sad to see a work of so much value – full of such useful information – disfigured by a few serious and elementary mistakes'.[9] In criticizing the statistics on which Miss Nightingale based her gloomy view of the work of hospitals, the reviewer noted that they were based on the *Report of the Registrar-General for 1861* and 'therefore, perhaps Miss Nightingale can hardly be held responsible for it'.[10] He continued:[11]

In 1861, returns were made from 106 Hospitals, giving the number of inmates in each on April 8. The number of deaths registered in each Hospital during the year 1861 is also given. Our readers will hardly believe that on these two bases a percentage of mortality is struck. The inmates of a single day are balanced with the deaths of a whole year, and no wonder the results are 'striking enough'. . . . There is something audacious in the last column of this table, where twenty-four London Hospitals are accredited with a mortality per cent on inmates of 90·84. No doubt it will be said this is the quotient of the figures employed; but we entirely deny their validity and the accuracy of the impression thus conveyed.

This damning criticism was refuted by William Farr, the Registrar-General, who thought that the method used admitted 'of no ambiguity'.[12] But this was not the end of the correspondence, for both T. Holmes and J. S. Bristowe continued the criticism of the method of calculation. The culmination of the correspondence was a devastating letter by Bristowe which appeared to admit of no answer:[13]

> If, out of a fixed population of 10,000 persons, 200 die in the course of a year, the mortality will be at the rate of 2 per cent. But, if, during this supposed year, these same 10,000 persons had been successively inmates of an institution with 2,000 beds and the 200 deaths had happened within the walls of this institution, the result would have been for the institution a death-rate of 10 per cent. And again, if these same 10,000 persons had been on similar conditions inmates of an institution with 1,000 beds, or of one with 500 beds, the mortality of these institutions would have become respectively 20 per cent and 40 per cent.

Bristowe finally crushed the Registrar-General in the concluding paragraph of this criticism:[14]

> If Dr. Farr had made his calculations about Hospitals in a tentative spirit, with the object of ascertaining whether they were likely to lead to any useful results, he would have acted in a way to which no exception could have been taken; if, when he had obtained his results, he had published them, and had at the same time pointed out clearly all their imperfections, and that, even had they been perfect they would still have afforded no test at all of the relative healthiness of Hospitals, but possibly some test of the relative severity of cases admitted into Hospitals, his labours might have been regarded as trivial, but no complaint could have been made; but when both he, and Miss Nightingale under his guidance, not only publish such results, but themselves draw from them the inference, and try to mislead others into the belief, that the unhealthiness of Hospitals is in proportion to Dr. Farr's death-rates of Hospitals, we are bound to protest against the whole matter as an unfounded and mischievous delusion.

Thus, the evidence used to support the pessimistic case, though of formidable repute, received a severe criticism at the time of its publication and the statistics presented in it are open to great doubt.

When considering the death-rate figures it should be remembered that:[15]

> the death-rate, instead of being the measure of a single influence on the health of hospitals, is in truth the sum of the

influences of an almost infinite number of causes, all of which require to be duly considered and allowed for before any useful comparison can be made.

What do the figures, as published by the hospitals, indicate as being their experience during the eighteenth and nineteenth centuries?[16]

Perhaps the first essayist of note in the field of political arithmetic, William Petty, recorded the experiences of the two royal institutions in London:[17]

> In the Hospital of St. Bartholomew in London there was sent out and cured in the year 1685, 1764 Persons, and there died out of the said Hospital 252.

> Moreover there were sent out and cured out of St. Thomas's Hospital 1523, and buried 209, that is to say there were cur'd in both Hospitals 3287, and buried 3748, of which number the 461 buried is less than eighth part.

As an appendix to the *Spittal Sermons* 'preach'd before the Right Honourable the Lord Mayor, the Court of Aldermen, and the Governors of the several Hospitals of the City of London, in St. Bridget's Church' on Easter Monday each year the royal institutions published the numbers treated during the previous year. Thus, for example, in the year ending Easter Monday, 1726, 3,564 patients were cured and 245 died at St Bartholomew's Hospital and at St Thomas's Hospital 4,873 were cured and 392 died.[18] For the year ending Easter Monday, 1735, of patients entering St Bartholomew's 4,803 were cured, while 316 died; and at St Thomas's for the same year the figures were 4,688 and 307 respectively.[19]

A review of the figures issued by the voluntary hospitals during the eighteenth and nineteenth centuries shows a consistent picture of relatively low mortality among patients – the impression of the hospitals killing more than they cured created by William Farr and Florence Nightingale being completely erroneous. However, the terms used in the reports of 'cured' and 'relieved' may not have meant what they do today.[20]

The Salisbury General Infirmary treated 66,455 in-patients and 132,185 out-patients from its opening on 2 May 1767 to the end of the hospital-year 1875–6. Of the in-patients 26,811 were claimed to be cured and 3,428 relieved, while 2,014 patients had died under its care, a death-rate of approximately 3 per cent.[21] In individual years the proportions did not appear to vary greatly, of 202 in-patients treated in 1770–1, 137 were cured, 5 relieved and only 6 died, a death-rate again of about 3 per cent.[22] In 1835–6, 627 were cured and 22 died out of 953 patients who completed their treatment in that year, a death-rate of nearly 2·5 per cent.[23]

From 1747 to 1846 the Salop Infirmary discharged 29,161 in-patients as cured and 21,096 as relieved. The deaths totalled 2,481 out of 56,819 completing their stay in the hospital, a death-rate of about 2·5 per cent.[24] Even when the figures are averaged over decade intervals the mortality-rates were still consistently low, thus from 1787 to 1796 there was an annual average of 27 deaths out of a total of 431 patients admitted each year. From 1827 to 1836 out of an annual average of 855 patients admitted 30 died.[25]

These figures are representative of the smaller provincial hospitals in the eighteenth and nineteenth centuries, and it is noticeable that even in the larger provincial and metropolitan hospitals the claimed mortality-rates were only a little higher.

As an illustration, at Manchester Infirmary in the year 1769–70 12 patients died and 16 were found to be incurable, but 286 were cured or relieved and 193 were made out-patients.[26] By the year 1874–5 a grand total of 1,522,504 patients had been treated, of which 959,346 were claimed to have been cured, 126,770 relieved and 49,744 had died.[27] The Bristol Infirmary generally exhibited mortality-rates of between 8 and 10 per cent annually; for example, figures of 8·4 per cent and 9·4 per cent were recorded in 1811 and 1828 respectively.[28] In the hospital-year 1760–1 at the Liverpool Infirmary, 207 in-patients were cured, 7 relieved and 12 died out of a total of 244 treated, a death-rate of approximately 5 per cent.[29] In 1875 the death-rate had risen to about 9 per cent, when 1,282 in-patients were cured, 615 relieved and 189 died out of a total of 2,086 treated at the same hospital.[30] For the Royal Infirmaries in Edinburgh and Glasgow the death-rates fluctuated from as low as 5 per cent to as high as 11 per cent.[31] St Thomas's Hospital in London showed the same sort of variation, rising from 7·25 per cent in the period 1786 to 1790 to 12·15 per cent in the period from 1870 to 1876.[32]

Improvements were made in hygiene and cleanliness at St Thomas's Hospital in 1783, and a comparison was made between the mortality in the ten preceding and ten subsequent years by its famous physician Sir Gilbert Blane:[33]

I found the former to be in the proportion of one to fourteen, the latter of 1 to 15·6. The average rate of mortality for the next ten years was 1 to 14·2; but in the last ten years, that is from 1803 till the present year, 1813, it has been 1 in 16·2. The average for the last fifty years, that is, from 1764, at which time the accounts of in-patients and out-patients were kept distinct, has been one in fifteen.

Another contemporary account reported that:[34]

In the great hospitals in London, of all admitted as in-patients about one in 13 died; in the Salop Infirmary, one in 11; in the Worcester Infirmary, one in 9; in the Old Northampton Infirmary, one in 14; and in the Newcastle Infirmary, one in 16: While, in the improved Hospital at Woolwich, only one in 35 dies; in the New Infirmary at Northampton, about one in 31; in the Leeds Infirmary, one in 28; and in the Infirmary at Glasgow, about one in 21; including infectious disease.

The first comprehensive analysis of hospital returns was made by the Rev. Oxenden in 1825, and he continued his studies in subsequent years for a number of government committees. His report on twenty-seven hospitals for the year 1830 showed that mortality varied from a low point of $2\frac{7}{17}$ per cent at Winchester County Hospital to a high point of $9\frac{3}{5}$ per cent at Bristol Infirmary. The general rate of mortality in the hospitals considered had a mean of approximately $4\frac{1}{2}$ per cent.[35]

The well-known collector of statistics, G. R. Porter, noted the variation in death-rates registered by different hospitals – 'That difference is no doubt capable of satisfactory explanation, for it would be absurd to suppose, that if the regulations and other circumstances attending the practice of different hospitals in the same city were the same, the rate of mortality should from year to year be so different'.[36] At St Bartholomew's Hospital he wrote that the rate of mortality in any period of five years from 1790 to 1834 had never been greater than 8·3 per cent and in those forty-four years the average was 7·53 per cent; and in the last five years of the series was only 7·25 per cent:[37]

whereas, in other general hospitals of this metropolis, which enjoy the advantage of medical and surgical skill on the part of their officers of St. Bartholomew's, the average rate of mortality has, in the same period of five years, exceeded 11 per cent;

being in the proportion of more than three deaths to two. On the other hand, the mortality during the last five years in the Infirmaries of Manchester and Liverpool has been even smaller than that of St. Bartholomew's Hospital: the average in the first-mentioned of these infirmaries proves to be 7·16 per cent, and that of Liverpool only 5·57 per cent.

The impression that mortality was lower in the smaller voluntary hospitals in the provinces than in those in the larger provincial towns is maintained by a survey made by a committee established by the Birmingham General Hospital in 1844. For the hospital-year 1841–2 three hospitals, the Bedford General Infirmary, the Suffolk General Infirmary (Bury St Edmunds), and the Gloucester Infirmary recorded death-rates of under 2 per cent. The Birmingham General Hospital itself and the Manchester Royal Infirmary recorded figures of 8·65 per cent and 8·12 per cent respectively.[38]

An interesting survey of the experiences of hospitals was published soon after the revelations of Miss Nightingale and William Farr. Though this study by Fleetwood Buckle completely refuted the statistics produced by the two illustrious figures of Miss Nightingale and Mr Farr, it has not received its due share of publicity, even at the time of its first appearance.[39] In 117 hospitals in England and Wales, which completed a questionnaire, 95,661 in-patients were treated in 1863, of which 7,361 died, a death-rate of 7·607 per cent. When this figure is broken down to its constituent parts, it is found that the eighteen metropolitan hospitals treated 53,031 in-patients and recorded a death-rate of 9·19 per cent; the 92 English provincial hospitals treated 59,681 in-patients and recorded a 7·672 per cent mortality-rate; and the 7 Welsh hospitals treated 12,524 in-patients and recorded the low death-rate of only 3·58 per cent.[40] When J. S. Bristowe and T. Holmes compiled their report in 1863 for the Medical Officer of the Privy Council, they found that again the death-rates recorded by hospitals were much lower than had been reported by Miss Nightingale and the Registrar-General – the highest figure found being 13·6 per cent at the Manchester Royal Infirmary.[41]

Some explanation is needed of the disparities in the death-rates between the voluntary hospitals and over time. An initial approach is to repeat the statement from the report of Bristowe and Holmes that the death-rate 'instead of being the measure of a single influence on the health of hospitals, is in truth the sum of the influences of an almost infinite number of causes, all of which require to be duly considered and allowed for before any useful comparison can be made'.[42] The categories used by the authors of the report will be taken as a basis for this analysis of the fate of patients who entered the voluntary hospitals.

The hospitals in London and in the large provincial centres of population were more likely to receive a greater proportion of accidents which were potentially more fatal than hospitals in rural areas. Even within London the experience of hospitals was different. Thus, the London Hospital in Whitechapel Road 'which is placed in the centre of one of the densest and poorest districts, and in close proximity to the Docks, and a large number of serious accidents than any other hospital in London',[43] recorded high death-rates. All the annual reports of this hospital remarked on this aspect of its work; for example, in the report for 1795 it was stated that 'Upwards of four hundred . . . were dreadful Casualties, as Fractures, Dislocations, Wounds, Scalds, &c. and extraordinary cases, received into the House without Recommendation'. Two hundred and eighteen persons were treated as out-patients and the total number treated in that year was 2,850.[44] In 1833 at the same hospital 972 accident cases were treated as in-patients out of a total of 2,517 admitted during that year,[45] and by 1863 the total of accident cases treated at the London Hospital had reached 12,488, of which 2,180 were admitted into the house.[46] In contrast, at Guy's Hospital in the same year only 4,704 accident cases were treated.[47]

The hospitals situated in the manufacturing towns had a similar problem. At the Sheffield Royal Infirmary it was stated for the year 1844–5 that '196 In-Patients, with sudden Accidents, &c., have been admitted during the past year without any recommendation; some of them with fractured limbs, and others with dislocations, wounds, contusions, burns and scalds'.[48] The accident cases were out of a total of 904 in-patients admitted during the year, of which 90 were still present at the end of the hospital-year.

The report of the Sheffield Royal Infirmary for the year 1844–5 was the prelude to increasing concern about the number of accident cases admitted into the hospital, and in 1848 a special report showed that on 9 February of that year at twelve-noon there were 106 patients in the house of which 30 were accident cases. Ten of the 30 accident patients were railway casualties which were proving to be increasingly prevalent.[49] In 1855 the state was reached whereby it was stated that 'An increased and increasing population, the proximity of railways, the continued introduction of complicated machinery, rendering accidents more frequent, tend continually to augment the necessity for a larger amount of accommodation in the Infirmary.'[50]

Even the smaller infirmaries were affected by growing industrialization and the spread of transport facilities. As an illustration, during the hospital-year 1845–6 no less than 67 accident cases were admitted to the wards of the Salisbury General Infirmary from the works on the Bishopstoke and Salisbury Railway.[51] But it needed a special incident of this kind before the small provincial hospitals felt a need to make mention of the accident cases admitted, while the larger metropolitan and provincial hospitals, such as the London Hospital, invariably published in their annual reports figures on the accident cases treated in each year.

The second influence on mortality in the voluntary hospital system to be considered is 'the pressure on the resources of hospitals in consequence of disproportion between the accommodation which they are capable of affording and the number of those applying for relief'.[52] This rather verbose statement can be defined more succinctly in terms of bed occupancy. The voluntary hospitals in London and the large provincial towns had the greatest turnover of patients as the demand for beds always appeared to exceed the supply available. Pleas were made continually either for extending hospital facilities or for a reduction in the privileges granted to subscribers to enable the larger hospitals to cope with the demand for their services. As an example in an important provincial town, Leeds, the General Infirmary reported in 1786 that 'During the two last Years, the average Number of In-Patients on the Books, waiting their turn for Admission into the House, has not been less than Twenty-five at a Time'.[53] This, undoubtedly, would have had effects on the time that a patient was allowed to convalesce after treatment in a hospital; though the cases likely to be admitted to hospitals in metropolitan or large provincial hospitals were usually of a more serious and acute character than those entering the smaller rural hospitals. J. S. Bristowe and T. Holmes, in their report, found that in four London hospitals the average number of patients per bed in 1862 was 10·9, in seven large provincial hospitals 10·6, and in fourteen rural hospitals 8·05. 'The extremes are the Liverpool Royal Infirmary, in which each bed has, in the course of a year, more than thirteen successive inmates, and the hospital at Colchester, where each bed has less than six.'[54]

The mortality attendant on surgical cases was less than that on medical cases and this was reflected in the overall mortality of a hospital by the proportion of each type of case, i.e. surgical or medical, admitted:[55]

> the great bulk of surgical cases consists of affections of the surface of the body, or of parts accessible from without, affections which are not of a lethal character or have only a remote tendency to a fatal issue. Indeed it frequently happens that almost the entire surgical mortality in a hospital depends on the deaths of the accident cases which have been admitted into it. . . . Medical cases, on the other hand, even if (as in many of the country hospitals) infectious diseases be excluded, always comprise, in addition to a varying degree of urgent cases, a large proportion of organic diseases of vital organs which necessarily tend directly, and often speedily, to a fatal result.

Thus, as illustrations, in 1862 at Guy's Hospital in London and at the Sheffield Royal Infirmary overall mortality was virtually identical at 9·61 per cent and 9·5 per cent respectively. The mortality in each hospital, in both the medical and the surgical cases, was again very similar; at Guy's the mortality was 14·49 per cent for medical cases and 6·16 per cent for surgical cases, while at the Sheffield Royal Infirmary the respective mortality figures were 14·6 per cent and 6·3 per cent.[56] At the Bristol Royal Infirmary for the same year the mortality in medical cases was 6·7 per cent and in surgical cases 3·7 per cent, giving an overall death-rate of 5·2 per cent. The total mortality at the Dundee Royal Infirmary was 7·0 per cent which was composed of a 10·7 per cent death-rate for medical cases and 3·0 per cent for surgical cases.[57] 'It is important to bear in mind that in almost all English hospitals a larger number of beds is allotted to the practice of surgery than to the practice of medicine, while . . . in most Scotch hospitals these proportions of medical and surgical beds are reversed.'[58] The Scottish hospitals usually allotted approximately two-thirds of their beds to medical cases, while in the English hospitals the balance was just in favour of the surgical cases. Thus, for example, the Hull Royal Infirmary in 1862 provided 54·9 per cent of the beds for surgical cases and 45·1 per cent[59] for medical cases:[60]

> Again, the admission or exclusion of cases of infectious diseases forms a very important item in regulating the mortality

of a hospital; and this is not merely because infectious diseases, such as typhus and small-pox, present normally a far larger percentage mortality than most other cases admitted into hospitals, but because practically, the admission or non-admission of this class of affections regulates in no small degree the admission of other acute medical diseases. . . . So that the hospital which declines to receive fever cases into its wards, ceases in large proportion to receive cases of acute internal inflammation which really form the great bulk of the urgent cases which physicians are called upon to treat.

Mortality from fever was subject to great fluctuation as at the London Fever Hospital from 1805 to 1876[61] when the death-rate varied from 9·0 per cent to 25·5 per cent:[62]

From the annual death register of the more important causes of death at Guy's, it would appear that the years 1741–42 contributed a larger number of fatal cases of fever than any others in the series, although later on in the century the deaths from the same cause spread over any given number of years maintained even a higher relative proportion than they did in the first half. . . . As new hospitals came to be founded, and better provision made for the poor in the workhouse infirmaries, the annual complement of fever cases in the London hospitals diminished, while from the growth of the population in other large towns, which, as a rule, were limited to but one hospital, the fever cases, especially in such as were liable to recurrent epidemics, greatly increased. This accounts partly for the increase of mortality during the present century in such hospitals as those situated in Manchester, Edinburgh, and Glasgow, and other towns where fever was treated either in the general wards or in separate wards of the respective hospitals.

This comment by the Superintendent of Guy's Hospital in the second half of the nineteenth century is illustrated by a comparison of the mortality-rates at the Glasgow and Edinburgh Royal Infirmaries for the period from 1808 to 1817 and 1866 to 1875. 'The mean death-rate during the first period was . . . 5·9 for the Edinburgh and 6·9 for the Glasgow Hospital, while in the more recent decade, it has preserved an average of 10·5 per cent in both institutions. But apart from fever, there were other agencies to account for a fluctuating death-rate.'[63] This last point is of great importance as, for example,

K

the Glasgow Royal Infirmary recorded an overall death-rate in 1862 of 10·3 per cent; 'but the death-rate in the fever wards was 16·7, and that of the hospital (excluding fever cases from computation) 8·7 only'.[64]

It was usually the practice of the voluntary hospitals to refuse admission to persons suffering from incurable diseases – 'Now such diseases include organic affections of the heart in their later stages, advanced Bright's disease, cancerous affections, and especially confirmed phthisis. It is notorious that the affections here enumerated . . . constitute the chief causes of death in those who have passed beyond the age of puberty.'[65] If phthisis, i.e. consumption, is considered at the Glasgow Royal Infirmary, the death-rate from this disease was 34·8 per cent from 1829 to 1832, which constituted 7·8 per cent of total deaths; 43·1 per cent from 1844 to 1849, constituting 14·0 per cent of total deaths; and 30·1 per cent from 1871 to 1876, constituting 16·6 per cent of total deaths.[66] A study of St Bartholomew's, St Thomas's and Guy's Hospitals and the Glasgow Royal Infirmary in the third quarter of the nineteenth century found that:[67]

> on an average 128 in every 1,000 patients are treated for diseases of the respiratory organs (cardiac diseases being excluded), that the death-rate among the phthisical has a mean of about 33 per cent, among other chest diseases 21 per cent, or taken together the gross mortality would amount to 25·3 per cent, or about 1 in 4 of the patients treated for chest affections.

However, many of the voluntary hospitals, particularly in the provincial towns and rural areas, adhered to the exclusion ruling:

> the Salop Infirmary, with 133 beds, and (in 1862) 1,030 admissions, presents for that year a death rate of 3·9% and among the deaths two only are ascribed to phthisis. Now, had the cases of phthisis formed a proportion of the whole number of cases admitted equal to that which obtains in St. Bartholomew's, St. Thomas's, or Guy's, the deaths due to this affection alone would have amounted to about 20, and the death rate would have been increased from 3·98 to 5·7.[68]

> Now in the London hospitals generally there is no rule tending to exclude dead or dying cases. . . . The same is the case as regards the hospitals of some of our large provincial towns, and in a few of those which go under the name of country

hospitals; but in the majority of these latter institutions the rule not only exists, but is enforced, and we have several times been informed by house surgeons (and the hospital records have for the most part amply confirmed such statements), that dying cases are really never admitted willingly into the wards.[69]

As support for this statement the authors found that at St Bartholomew's Hospital one-sixth of all mortality could be accounted for by patients either being brought dead to the hospital or dying within twenty-four hours of admission. This was a problem which faced many of the provincial hospitals, particularly among those which admitted fever cases:[70]

Besides the obvious inhumanity of this procedure, it is to be remarked that the reception of moribund cases greatly swells the number of deaths recorded as occuring in the Hospital, and very materially increases the proportionate mortality thereby producing misconceptions in the public mind, as to the comparative advantages of treating Epidemic diseases in public Hospitals, and in the dwellings of the poor.

An illustration of this can be seen at the Manchester Royal Infirmary, where in the hospital-year 1860–1 of the 293 deaths recorded out of 2,001 in-patients admitted to the hospital, 183 were said to be dying at the time of their admission.[71]

If a hospital admits a large proportion of such ailments as venereal diseases, eye diseases and skin diseases where the prospects of a fatal termination are remote, the mortality-rate of such a hospital will be less than that of a hospital which does not admit such cases. Thus, at Guy's Hospital in 1862, 395 eye cases were admitted, none of which proved fatal.[72] The provision of special wards for patients suffering from venereal disease did not mean necessarily that all the beds were in constant use if letters of recommendation had to be obtained for admittance. This was the case, for example, at the Chester Infirmary; but at the Liverpool Infirmary in 1802 it was stated that in future years preference would have to be given to venereal patients from the town and its immediate vicinity as the capacity of the wards was not sufficient to cope with the numbers requesting admission from a distance.[73] Some of the voluntary hospitals developed a speciality in one form of disease and as a result admitted a large number of cases of that particular type. The Devon and Exeter Hospital found that a large percentage of cases admitted were for skin diseases as the physicians of that hospital had acquired a reputation for treating skin affections.[74]

With regard to 'trivial cases':[75]

> The admission or exclusion of trivial cases, by which we mean
> (on the physician's side of the hospital) chronic dyspepsia,
> incipient phthisis, hypochondriasis, hysteria, amenorrhoea,
> 'debility', and a number of nervous and other disorders which
> frequently come under the care of the medical practitioner, but
> to which names can scarcely be assigned, and (on the surgical
> side) ulcerated legs, varicose veins, chronic joint affections not
> demanding operation, trivial injuries, such as cut and broken
> fingers, and the like – the admission or exclusion of such cases
> as these unquestionably forms one of the great distinctions
> between the hospitals of large towns and those which are
> usually termed country hospitals . . . admissions limited to
> special days, and especially the plan of admission by
> governor's letters, tend (especially in rural hospitals), to fill the
> hospital beds with chronic or trivial cases, which are retained
> in the house, not for any actual benefit they are likely to
> receive, but out of deference to the recommendations which
> secured their admission.

Many of the voluntary hospitals provided facilities for a number of pupils of the physicians and surgeons from which, in the nineteenth century, medical schools developed.[76] A different type of patient was attracted to these hospitals than to those which did not have teaching facilities:[77]

> The effect flowing not absolutely from skilful treatment, but
> from the reputation of a hospital, and from the interest taken
> in their duties by members of the hospital staff . . . undoubtedly
> exerts what may be termed a very unfavourable influence
> indeed over the death rate. . . . A hospital which enjoys a high
> reputation has, in addition to the serious cases it attracts
> normally from a limited area, numerous selected cases, of a
> serious nature, habitually transmitted to it by medical men
> (old pupils and others) residing at a distance.

This was particularly noticeable in the larger teaching institutions, especially in the metropolitan hospitals, the Edinburgh and Glasgow Royal Infirmaries, and the General Infirmary at Leeds.

These influences on the mortality prevalent in hospitals, as expressed by J. S. Bristowe and T. Holmes, help to explain the wide variations between different hospitals, particularly between the rural and the town hospitals. The differences in the death-rates were used by the protagonists concerned with the salubrity of hospitals to demonstrate that the hospitals in the country were far safer for the patients than those situated in urban areas. This controversy raged during the middle years of the nineteenth century and the report to the Privy Council by Dr J. S. Bristowe and T. Holmes was an attempt to bring a little reason to the debate.[78] They stated that:[79]

The general death-rates of hospitals afford no test of the relative salubrity of hospitals. The condition of a hospital death-rate is determined almost exclusively by the character of the cases admitted, and by the rules or the practices which regulate their discharge. The variations of death-rate due to hospital insalubrity are confined within very narrow limits, and are wholly or almost wholly lost among the far greater variations dependent on the conditions referred to. . . . English rural hospitals have acquired, on false grounds, a reputation for comparative healthiness. By their regulations, their practice, or their position, they receive habitually a far less serious class of cases than is admitted into the hospitals of London and other large towns. This difference in the quality of the practice is much greater in respect of medicine than of surgery, but is considerable even as regards surgery. The result is marked lowness of death-rate even (in many cases) in the presence of a high degree of hospital insalubrity.

An alternative method of analysing the effectiveness of hospitals is to study the mean length of stay of patients admitted. It would be reasonable to assume that as the practice of medicine developed and became more refined the length of stay would be diminished, though this would be offset by the developments in medicine allowing more complex cases to be treated. If the Salop Infirmary is taken as an example of a provincial hospital, the reduction in the number of days a patient stayed in the hospital can be seen clearly. In its first decade (1747 to 1756) the Salop Infirmary recorded a mean residence of 94 days; this subsequently diminished to 44 days in the period from 1777 to 1786; and fell further to 36 days in the decade from 1837 to 1846.[80] In the hospital-year of 1830 the Leicester Infirmary found that its patients remained within the house for an average of just over 28 days; while the Gloucester Infirmary, at the other extreme, needed 101 days, on average, to complete the treatment of its patients. A crude average length of stay for 21 provincial hospitals for this year was calculated at 43 days.[81] A calculation made for the hospital-year 1863 found that in 177 hospitals in England and Wales the average length of stay was 32·32 days, the average in the 110 hospitals in England alone was 35·25 days. In the 18 metropolitan hospitals the average length of stay was recorded as 32·17 days, and in the 92 English provincial hospitals as 34·42 days.[82]

An attempt has recently been made to make a more accurate estimate of the average length of stay according to the type of voluntary hospital, using the material found in the work of Fleetwood Buckle and in the report prepared by Bristowe and Holmes.[83] For the year 1861[84] the study, covering 87 per cent of the beds in teaching hospitals and 59 per cent of those in general hospitals, finds that the average length of stay in the teaching hospitals was 33·5 days and in the general hospitals 40·6 days, giving a combined average of 36·2 days.[85] A comparison of the London and the provincial teaching hospitals shows that there was little difference in the average length of stay, being 33·3 days and 33·8 days respectively.[86] However:[87]

> There was a far wider range of averages within the provincial general group. For example, the average length of stay at the Bath Royal United was 27·3 days, while at the Essex and Colchester it was 62·7 days and at the South Devon and East Cornwall the average was nearly 70 days.

A further breakdown of the figures for the London and the Provincial teaching hospitals shows that there was a far greater variance in the averages in the provinces than in London.[88]

> The lowest London average was in the Royal Free (24·5 days), which with only 84 beds was the smallest of the metropolitan teaching hospitals. The highest average – 38 days – was that of St. Thomas's. . . . [In the provinces] the lowest average of 27·9 days at the Liverpool Royal Infirmary may be compared with the highest average of 48·9 days at the Radcliffe Infirmary, Oxford. The average of Addenbrooke's Hospital, Cambridge, was only slightly lower at 44·7 days. A third provincial establishment with an average in excess of 40 days was the Royal Victoria Infirmary, Newcastle. Thus in 1861 three of the eight provincial teaching hospitals were keeping

their patients longer than the average provincial general hospital of that year.

A study of two typical provincial hospitals, one in England and the other in Scotland, shows a similar pattern for the period after 1861. From 1864 to 1874 the average length of stay at the Hull Royal Infirmary fluctuated about a 30-day mean. The lowest figure of 29 days was recorded in 1870 and the highest of 34 days was recorded twice in the year 1866 and 1873. The length of stay was longer for surgical cases than for medical cases, being 37 days and 31 days respectively in 1873.[89] These figures are borne out by the experience of the Scottish hospital, the Glasgow Royal Infirmary, which, in 1875, recorded an average residence of $32\frac{1}{2}$ days – the average stay for medical patients being $28\frac{1}{2}$ days, that for surgical cases $37\frac{1}{2}$ days, and 25 days for fever patients.[90]

Although: 'Duration of stay in hospital is determined practically by such various circumstances, is so dependent on the caprice of medical attendants, so dependent on the rules of hospitals, on the pressure of applicants for admission, and on the nature of the cases received that . . . [it] becomes of little value as a test of anything',[91] the conclusions reached by Bristowe and Holmes in their report appear to fit the information which is available. They concluded that 'patients remain longer in country than in town hospitals; that the stay of surgical patients exceeds in duration that of medical patients; and that acute affections, such as fevers, remain under treatment for a shorter time than other forms of medical disease'.[92]

Although mortality in voluntary hospitals was not unduly high, consideration must be given to the method used in the compilation of the figures and to the possibility of 'adjustment'. The voluntary hospitals were dependent on financial support from private individuals and success had to be seen if subscriptions were to be maintained and new ones encouraged. The figures used to calculate the death-rate prevailing in a hospital could be adjusted in a number of ways. Bristowe and Holmes wrote:[93]

> in the majority of hospitals, it is we believe, the custom to reckon among their deaths those who have been brought dead to the institution; but there are many hospitals where such cases are not reckoned, and there are some indeed where even those who die within 24 hours are, on the ground that they were moribund at the time of admission, excluded from computation.

In the annual reports of the voluntary hospitals such cases were listed under a separate category and allowance has been made for these cases in the calculations used. A large percentage of the deaths in the larger metropolitan and provincial hospitals was provided by this category, and if these cases were excluded from the compilation of the returns a considerable improvement in the death-rate recorded could be engineered.

A more serious charge which could be levied against a hospital would be the proposition that it discharged a patient as death appeared to be imminent, thereby removing a potential death from its records. An example of this occurrence may have happened at the Radcliffe Infirmary, Oxford, in 1786. The case was reported in the local newspaper:[94]

> on Saturday last an inquest was taken . . . on view of the body of Ann Jutt, a poor woman, who was discharged from our Infirmary on the Thursday preceding and who had not walked from the House more than a hundred yards before she dropped down dead. The Jurors' verdict was that she died by the visitation of God.

This may well have been a correct verdict as even today patients have been known to be discharged from a hospital in a seemingly fit state who collapse and die from some previously undiagnosed cause shortly after. In the eighteenth and, indeed, the nineteenth centuries when diagnosis was imperfect there is more reason to believe that these episodes may have occurred. However, the practice of dismissal must have been known, for a Dundee surgeon, commenting on the success of his operations in the local infirmary in 1842, said that it was in no way due to 'any urging of patients to leave the house when they were found to be approaching a fatal termination, a mode by which a medical attendant of an hospital at any time, may bring the mortality to a convenient ratio'.[95] Bristowe and Holmes pointed out:[96]

> Again, in many hospitals it is the practice to specify in the reports the total number of cases under treatment during the year, including in this phrase not only those who were actually admitted, but those cases (admitted in the previous year) that were in the wards at the commencement of the hospital year. To this, of course, no one can object, but it happens and not very infrequently, that the death-rate is calculated on this total

number of cases under treatment, instead of being calculated on the admissions alone, or on (what is yet more correct) the cases treated to a termination.

Robert Lawson Tait found that in 'this way a number of patients are reckoned twice, and . . . that in some hospitals it made a difference of nearly ten per cent of the whole returns'.[97]

> Further, there is another practice, still more pernicious, which we know is far from uncommon. It is that of giving to patients, after they have been six weeks or two months in hospital, renewed tickets and counting them from that time as new admissions. . . . Thus in one instance, out of 626 nominal patients no less than 169 were duplicates. Including this latter number in the computation the death rate was 4·7 excluding this number it mounted up to 6·5.[98]

This device and the one described in the previous paragraph 'sometimes made a difference of one per cent on the patient death-rate for the decade – of course, in favour of the hospital'.[99] It is difficult to check the extent of this practice, although in the annual reports of some voluntary hospitals the number of 'renewed' patients was declared. For example, the annual report of the Leicester Infirmary in 1870 stated that the institution had treated a total of 1,682 in-patients, of which 166 were classified under the category of 'renewed recommendations'.[100] In 1875 at the same hospital it was stated that there were 154 such 'renewed recommendations'.[101] Therefore, when any calculation is made of the death-rate in a voluntary hospital the patients in this category can be excluded:[102]

> There are other modes of falsification which imply actual dishonesty, but which we believe to be very rarely practised, and which consequently can have no appreciable influence on the death-rate. Thus in one institution which shall be nameless, we were assured that one of the surgeons had been known, in a case of operation about to end fatally, to take down the original ticket, and to supply the patient with a new one, in order that the case might be counted as two, viz. first a case of successful operation, and second, a case of death from erysipelas, or whatever the immediate cause of death may have been. We give this statement as we receive it, but do not pledge ourselves as to its truth.

To add to these qualifications about the compilation of the statistics provided by the voluntary hospitals Robert Lawson Tait wrote that when he attempted to compare the death-rate against the average length of stay he 'found the same tendency to exaggeration here, for it was not an unusual thing to find a hospital returning two or three times the number of beds which it could, by any possibility, have in actual use'.[103]

Although these objections to the compilation of the statistics could prove serious in any computation of the death-rate or the average length of stay, most of them can be discovered and allowance made for them. The only malpractice which would be difficult to take account of would be the removal of a patient before his expected death. However, as the voluntary hospitals were dependent on subscriptions success and respectability had to be demonstrated, and such a practice would have very quickly brought a hospital into disrepute. The practice would have become common knowledge through the local newspaper, as at the Radcliffe Infirmary at Oxford, and if it was repeatedly put into effect the resultant publicity would have been more than the hospital could have borne without damage to its reputation.

Thus, the conclusions to be reached about the experience of the voluntary hospitals during the eighteenth and nineteenth centuries, even making allowances for 'adjustment', are favourable towards their contribution to the health of the community. The hospitals did achieve what appears to be a remarkable degree of success in treating their patients and the mortality remained at a low level throughout the period, generally being under 10 per cent of the patients admitted.

the chief indictment of hospital work at this period is not that it did no good, but that it positively did harm. . . . The common cause of death was infectious disease; any patient admitted to hospital faced the risk of contracting a mortal infection . . . it was not until much later [than the eighteenth century] that hospital patients could be reasonably certain of dying from the disease with which they were admitted.[1]

In such words the contribution of hospitals in the period under consideration has been condemned by two eminent medical historians. Such statements by acknowledged experts have been taken over by economic and social historians who, afraid to venture into unknown territory, have accepted the above view with little thought or criticism. This can be seen in the contributions made by historians to the continuing debate on the nature of British population growth in the eighteenth and early nineteenth centuries. 'Hospitals . . . were more likely to spread disease than to check it. People who went to hospital in the eighteenth century normally died there, generally from some disease other than that with which they were admitted.'[2] 'There is . . . no evidence at all that eighteenth century hospitals did improve their patients' chances of survival. They were hot-beds of infection so that the danger of mortality rose when a patient entered one.'[3] Indeed, one historian has been moved to describe hospitals in the eighteenth century as being 'gateways to death'.[4]

The evidence presented by medical historians has given the voluntary hospitals a formidable reputation, thereby denying that medical improvements could have assisted in any way in a reduction in the death-rate of the community during the eighteenth century. In fact, the thesis is taken further and it is argued that not only were changes in medical facilities not resulting in falling mortality, but that they may have well contributed to an increase in mortality.

The records of the voluntary hospitals concerning the fate of their patients suggest that the 'pessimistic' view may need to be reappraised. Hospitals were not 'gateways to death'. Although conditions in hospitals were of a very low standard, compared with the present day, the death-rate was generally low. This can be ascribed to the rules of admission which excluded the 'problem' cases, and to the small amount of operative surgery performed which minimized the likelihood of sepsis. The outbreaks of 'hospital diseases' which did occur had only a marginal effect on overall hospital mortality. This revision of the experience of the voluntary hospitals suggests some re-examination of their contribution to the health of the community.

The numbers treated by the voluntary hospitals as in-patients appear to have been comparatively small; though, of course, the hospitals also treated a considerable number of out-patients. The voluntary hospital system provided treatment which would otherwise not have been available, the provision of beds rising from approximately 4,000 in 1800 to approximately 12,000 in England and Wales in 1861. A very substantial increase, when at the beginning of the eighteenth century there were only the two royal institutions of St Bartholomew's and St Thomas's in London.

As a proportion of the total population the number of patients treated in the voluntary hospitals was minimal, being in the region of 30,000 in-patients in 1801 when there were approximately 10 million people in England, Wales and Scotland. However, the number of people who were potential patients in the voluntary hospitals was limited. The hospitals were established principally in the capital and in the main provincial centres of population so that the bed provision was concentrated in the areas most likely to make use of a hospital's services. Their facilities were restricted to that part of the population known as the 'labouring' or 'deserving' poor. For the poor the voluntary hospitals provided their sole means of formal medical treatment, other than the apothecaries and quacks, as they were generally unable to afford the services of the physicians and surgeons who were in private practice.[5] If the treatment provided by the voluntary hospitals for their patients was relatively successful, in that only a small percentage of those admitted died in the hospitals, then the contribution of the voluntary hospitals may have been favourable to the mortality of the community.

However, the nature of the demographic data available to the historian for the eighteenth century makes this an impossible task to achieve. If it were possible to establish control groups, i.e. two areas with similar characteristics of population composition, environment, etc., but one area possessing a voluntary hospital and the other not; then a comparison could be made between the death-rates prevailing in each area and any difference could be attributed to the absence or presence of a voluntary hospital. The only evidence relating to deaths from disease during the eighteenth century is that to be gained from the Bills of Mortality. These abstracts from the parish registers were begun to contrast normal levels of mortality with those of the plague. The Bills of Mortality, however, have been subject to considerable criticism, particularly in the method of collection, and as a result they do not have the accuracy necessary for serious demographic study.[6] An illustration of their unreliability is that in London in the middle of the eighteenth century no less than sixty-five burial places, accounting for about 10 per cent of all London burials, had not been taken account of in the Bills of Mortality.[7] Nevertheless, a study of the Bills of Mortality for Norwich suggested that 'the fall in mortality rates apparent in Norwich after 1760 would appear to have been related to some extent to the provision of improved medical facilities, environmental improvements of a relatively minor kind possibly providing some degree of reinforcement'.[8]

There are a number of further difficulties in assessing the contribution of the voluntary hospitals to population growth in the eighteenth century in that there were significant developments in other forms of medical treatment. As a complement to the work of the hospitals a network of dispensaries was established, also on a voluntary basis. These dispensaries provided medical services which the voluntary hospitals were unable or unwilling to give. 'Dispensaries are adapted to the cure not only of all chronic and such acute complaints as are uninfectious, but also of epidemic and contagious diseases, when raging (as among the poor is often the case) in the most violent and destructive manner.'[9] By 1802 it has been estimated that dispensaries were assisting 50,000 poor patients annually in the London area alone.[10] These institutions were probably important also in spreading knowledge about hygiene and sanitation, for one of the foremost physicians of the second half of the eighteenth century, John Lettsom, commented that 'In the space of a very few years I have observed a total revolution in the conduct of the common people respecting their diseased friends, they have learned that most diseases are mitigated by a free admission of air, by cleanliness and by promoting instead of retaining the indulgence and care of the sick'.[11]

A further development was the introduction of inoculation against smallpox, one of the endemic diseases of the eighteenth century. It has been suggested that after the improved method of inoculation was perfected by the Sutton brothers in the 1760s, it 'could theoretically explain the whole of the increase in population'.[12] Perhaps this statement is too sweeping, but it does illustrate the problem of separating the influences, good or bad, of changes in medical facilities and techniques on population growth in the eighteenth century.

However, despite the difficulties involved in assessing these changes during the eighteenth and early nineteenth centuries, it is possible to make a tentative conclusion about the role of the voluntary hospital system in the health of the community. The thesis that the voluntary hospitals may well have contributed to an increase in mortality, based as it is on extremely unreliable or irrelevant data, does not appear to be substantiated when the records of the individual hospitals are examined. Yet, having dismissed the 'pessimistic' view, it is not so easy to make a positive statement and suggest that the voluntary hospitals assisted a fall in mortality as the nature of the demographic data for the period does not allow any meaningful analysis to be made, either over time or between regions.[13]

This study of the records of the voluntary hospitals and of the contemporary literature has provided some new evidence about these institutions and it would seem reasonable to put forward the proposition that the miserable reputation that they have endured has little foundation. The voluntary hospitals may not have been the most hygienic or the most pleasant of institutions by the standards of today; nor may the standard of medical care have been very high; but they provided a service for a section of the population which had previously been neglected with some degree of success, and historians should judge them accordingly.

Appendix 1   The voluntary hospitals of the eighteenth century

English Hospitals

(a) London   *Date of opening*

Westminster Hospital	1720
Guy's Hospital	1724
St George's Hospital	1733
London Hospital	1740
Middlesex Hospital	1745

In addition there were two general chartered institutions:

St Bartholomew's Hospital	1123 (refounded 1546)
St Thomas's Hospital	1213 (refounded 1551)

(b) Provinces

Winchester County Hospital	1736
Bristol Royal Infirmary	1737
York County Hospital	1740
Royal Devon and Exeter Hospital	1741
Bath General Hospital	1742
Northampton General Hospital	1743
Worcester Royal Infirmary	1746
Royal Salop Infirmary	1747
Liverpool Royal Infirmary	1749
Royal Victoria Infirmary, Newcastle	1751
Manchester Royal Infirmary	1752
Gloucester Royal Infirmary	1755
Chester Infirmary	1755
Addenbrooke's Hospital, Cambridge	1766
Salisbury County Hospital	1766
Staffordshire County Hospital	1766
General Infirmary at Leeds	1767
Lincoln County Hospital	1769
Radcliffe Infirmary, Oxford	1770
Norfolk and Norwich Hospital	1771

Leicester Royal Infirmary	1771
Hereford General Infirmary	1776
Birmingham General Hospital	1779
Nottingham General Hospital	1782
Hull Royal Infirmary	1782
Bath City Infirmary	1792
Kent and Canterbury Hospital	1793
Sheffield Royal Infirmary	1797

Scottish Hospitals

	Date of opening
Edinburgh Royal Infirmary	1729
Aberdeen Royal Infirmary	1742
Dumfries and Galloway Royal Infirmary	1778
Glasgow Royal Infirmary	1792
Dundee Royal Infirmary	1798

In addition to the voluntary hospitals which were founded in the eighteenth century there were a number of dispensaries established, many of which expanded to form hospitals in the nineteenth century.

Appendix 2   An account of the establishment of the county hospital at Winchester*

As the Papers which have already been dispersed will not come into every body's hands, the Governors think it will be of use to lay before the Public in One view the many advantages of Hospitals in general; as well as an Account of the rise, progress and management of That which has been lately established here, and is the First of the kind that has been attempted in any part of the Kingdom except in London and Westminster.

They are glad to find, by the Spirit which their Example has raised in many places, that their Countrymen are at length awakened to a sense of the benefits of a Charity which is the most general, as well as unexceptionable of all others. And the certain experience they have had of every particular in a County that is thin of people, and has no settled Manufacture, must be a sufficient encouragement to Those who live in populous places, and amongst multitudes of distressed objects, to make the experiment: For an equal resolution will assuredly produce every where an equal effect, and defeat all attempts that can be made by men of narrow or selfish views to oppose an Establishment which will be of more use in the Country, than even in London, where every other help is always at hand.

1. It is the only certain way of relieving the Poor-Sick; who are frequently neglected and over-looked at their own Homes; because Physicians and Surgeons can neither give their attendance, nor dispense their Medicines with any convenience at more places than One, and because their concerns are of too private a nature to engage the attention of any but the very Few Who make it their business to inquire after Them.

2. It is the most safe and eligible manner of doing it; because the care and neatness, as well as the simplicity and regularity of Diet, with which the Poor are kept in an Hospital, do all contribute much sooner to their Recovery, than their own way of living; and are often

* Source: Winchester County Hospital, *An Account of the Establishment o, the County-Hospital at Winchester, with the Proceedings of the Governors, &c. from the first Institution on St. Luke's Day, October 18, 1736, to Michaelmas, 1737.*

more effectual than Physic in the Cure of Several of the most inveterate Distempers.

3. The Expence of relieving a great number of Sick Persons in an Hospital, bears no proportion to that of assisting them at their separate Homes: And the Widow's Mite entrusted with Those who can dispose of it to the utmost advantage, will go farther towards answering the Ends of Charity, than a Sum of Money bestowed at random on such as are incompetent judges of the use of it, or of the proper manner of laying it out.

4. It opens a Channel for private Charities which has been long wanted, and enables persons to lay them out to certain advantage; because Every One has it in his power from the moment he subscribes, to recommend a Patient, and by that means, may be assured, that his Bounty cannot be misapplied: Whereas almost all private Charities have hitherto been wasted, and rendered ineffectual thro' indolence, or want of knowing how to direct the expence; or by the various sorts of Mismanagement, which are in some measure unavoidable, and which are too well known, and too heavily felt, to need any particular explanation.

5. It is incapable of being so far abused or misapplied, as to make Any One repent of their Bounty; which will appear to Those Who consider that, tho' the greatest part of the income should really be perverted, there would still be more good done by it, than by a larger Sum in any other manner. For a thousand persons will be relieved here at a less expence, than would be required for an hundred in the ordinary way of giving Alms.

6. It is a Charity that is subject to no Imposture, but what must be discovered by the Physicians and Surgeons.

7. It prevents most of the Evils that are common to the Poor, by administring a present support in the time of Sickness; and does in some measure supply all their Wants more effectually than Money; for Money itself cannot provide that instant Relief which is here always at hand, and gives the Poor (in the case of Accidents, to which they are more subject) a considerable advantage over their Betters: The Supplies, that are immediately wanted, are here granted in kind without any delay. Advice and Medicines are to the Sick, what Food is to the Hungry, and Clothes to the Naked.

8. It provides for the relief and comfort of Multitudes who are unable to be at the expence of Advice or Physick, but are not distinguished by the name of The Poor, because They do not come under the care of a Parish or a Workhouse; and yet are the principal

objects of this Charity, and most of all entitled to the regards of the Public; since They are in present want; and are of the diligent and industrious, that is, of the useful and valuable part of all Society.

9. It multiplies every Good that can be done to the Poor in any other way, by easing whole Families of the burden of attending and providing for their sick Relations; so that the Miserable are relieved and comforted, and their Families are at liberty to earn their own Support at the same time.

10. It preserves Them from the ill usage of ignorant Quacks and Imposters Who too often take advantage of their Necessities; and not only insensibly drain them of the little Money Them have under pretence of selling cheap Medicines; but frequently destroy their Health for want of Honesty or Skill.

11. It is of infinite Use to All Other persons as well as the Poor, by furnishing the Physicians and Surgeons with more experience in one Year, than They could have in ten without it.

12. It is a most certain means of increasing the number of the People; as well as of saving a multitude of Hands, who are often lost for want of timely assistance: And it deserves to be remembered, that a third part of what every labouring Man earns, is so much clear gains to the Public.

13. It encourages Parishes (when They are relieved of the great burden of supporting the Sick) to provide better for the maintenance of Orphans and Aged Persons. And it is certain, that the number of both these sorts must gradually decrease, by a provident care of the Sick; Who will be enabled for the most part to educate their Children, as well as to provide beforehand for their own Support against the Extremities of Old Age.

14. It reduces the number of Vagrants by depriving them of one of their most plausible Reasons for begging from door to door, under the specious pretence of sick Relations or Friends for whom They are concerned: So that they who are Idle and able to work, will be obliged to have recourse to some Employment, and make themselves serviceable Members of the Community, when they are not supplied in the usual manner from the public and private Charities, which are too often distributed without any due regard to the different Necessities of the Poor.

15. It must have the strongest tendency to promote a Spirit of Religion and Virtue amongst the Common People; which by degrees may recover them out of that profligate State of Life which is the general complaint of these Times, and of the utmost consequence

to the Well-being of the whole Kingdom. The most certain method of recovering Men from their evil Courses, is to remove them out of the way of bad examples for so long a time as is necessary to beget contrary Habits. And it may be reasonably presumed that great numbers of the Poor will be insensibly reclaimed by the exact regularity of Manners, which is maintained in an Hospital as well as by the frequency of such Reflections as are naturally suggested in the House of Mourning. They are provided here with the use of the best Books, and have daily opportunities of being instructed by Those, whose Duty it is to attend upon this very thing. And as an Hospital is supplied with Patients from all parts, it must needs be, that a Spirit of Religion and Gratitude will be gradually spread throughout a whole Country. For We can never hope to secure their Affections, soften their Passions, reform their Manners, and possess them with a sense of their Duty to God and Their Superiors so effectually as by this feeling way to Instruction.

16. It is the most comprehensive of all Charities; because there is scarce any One Species of doing good which is not promoted by it. For the Sick are visited and relieved; the Stranger is taken in; the Ignorant instructed; the Bad reclaimed; present Wants are supplied, and future ones prevented; and (by easing Families of the burden of supporting their sick Friends) it is also a Means of feeding the Hungry, clothing the Naked, cherishing the industrious Poor, and preserving a multitude of useful Members to the Public Etc. Etc.

These are the Benefits which without any shadow of doubt are peculiar to this Charity, and are of great consequence to All and Singular; to the Rich as well as the Poor; and to the public as well as the private Estate of Men. Any One of them should be sufficient to convince Us of its use, and All of them together must warm Men into proper resolutions of encouraging and supporting a Charity, which is the Glory of other Countries and has long been the Reproach of Our Own.

Appendix 3 Mortality in selected voluntary hospitals to 1875

Table A3.1   Small provincial – Salisbury General Infirmary*

Year	Cured	Relieved	Other	Dead	In house	Total	Mortality %
2 May 1767– 1 Sept 1767	9	—	14	3	17	43	1·2
1 Sept 1770– 1 Sept 1771	137	5	67	6	13	228	2·8
1 Sept 1775– 1 Sept 1776	199	23	76	3	43	344	1·0
1 Sept 1780– 31 Aug 1781	260	25	64	12	37	398	3·3
30 Aug 1785– 31 Aug 1786	204	30	60	9	39	342	3·0
30 Aug 1790– 31 Aug 1791	198	15	110	9	34	366	2·7
30 Aug 1795– 31 Aug 1796	215	11	129	17	19	391	4·6
30 Aug 1800– 31 Aug 1801	259	31	110	7	23	430	1·7
30 Aug 1805– 31 Aug 1806	250	7	178	13	24	472	2·9
31 Aug 1810– 31 Aug 1811	183	23	212	7	26	451	1·6
31 Aug 1815– 31 Aug 1816	236	22	183	12	47	500	2·6
31 Aug 1820– 31 Aug 1821	315	8	222	6	37	588	1·1
31 Aug 1825– 31 Aug 1826	379	23	284	14	82	782	2·0
31 Aug 1830– 31 Aug 1831	436	2	365	16	69	888	2·0
31 Aug 1835– 31 Aug 1836	627	10	376	22	82	1,117	2·1

Table A3.1　Small provincial – Salisbury General Infirmary* (cont.)

Year	Cured	Relieved	Other	Dead	In house	Total	Mortality %
31 Aug 1840– 31 Aug 1841	274	11	632	21	99	1,037	2·2
23 Aug 1845– 22 Aug 1846	313	17	284	23	79	716	3·6
26 Aug 1850– 25 Aug 1851	202	34	599	34	96	965	3·9
26 Aug 1855– 31 July 1856	129	14	659	37	61	900	4·4
31 July 1860– 29 July 1861	211	104	482	19	65	881	2·3
27 July 1865– 28 July 1866	241	93	536	34	63	967	3·8
31 July 1870– 29 July 1871	215	87	650	33	60	1,045	3·4
31 July 1875– 29 July 1876	121	63	429	38	69	720	5·8

* Source: *Annual Reports.*

Table A3.2　Large provincial – Hull Royal Infirmary*

Year	Cured	Relieved	Other	Dead	In house	Total	Mortality %
26 Sept 1782– 1 Aug 1783	25	8	67	9	8	117	8·3
1 Aug 1784– 31 Dec 1785	129	21	21	20	20	211	10·5
1790	69	12	72	14	31	198	8·4
1795	128	21	33	8	24	214	4·2
1800	135	27	42	14	32	250	6·4
1805	153	21	43	5	56	278	2·3
1810	119	40	32	19	30	240	9·0
1815	148	51	51	16	40	306	6·0
1820	161	57	55	23	41	337	7·8
1825	172	66	57	19	41	355	6·1
1830	273	85	81	15	63	517	3·3
1835	322	80	85	32	77	596	6·2
1840	467	132	126	67	95	887	8·5

Table A3.2   Large provincial–Hull Royal Infirmary* (cont.)

Year	Cured	Relieved	Other	Dead	In house	Total	Mortality %
1845	497	122	89	46	81	835	6·1
1850	404	37	236	49	76	802	6·7
1855	508	77	106	35	110	836	4·8
1860	565	34	282	69	120	1,070	7·3
1865	680	181	159	77	107	1,204	7·0
1870	708	196	95	96	114	1,209	8·8
1875	851	—	82	95	82	1,110	9·2

* Source: *Annual Reports.*

Table A3.3   Large provincial – Manchester Royal Infirmary*

Year	Cured	Relieved	Other†	Dead	In house	Total	Mortality %
24 June 1752–24 June 1753	42	7	10	3	13	75	4·8
1754–5	89	14	32	9	44	188	6·3
1759–60	166	55	78	18	58	375	5·7
1764–5	192	52	138	16	79	477	4·0
1769–70	246	40	231	12	47	576	2·3
1774–5	224	46	196	23	72	561	4·7
1779–80	258	31	150	20	45	504	4·4
1784–5	258	31	159	11	73	532	2·4
1789–90	259	57	253	15	78	662	2·6
1794–5	365	33	318	41	72	829	5·4
1799–1800	355	21	323	30	75	804	4·1
1804–5	339	29	332	36	82	818	4·9
1809–10	421	60	325	28	69	903	3·4
1814–15	547	34	465	45	89	1,180	4·1
1819–20	500	30	564	72	84	1,250	6·2
1824–5	415	65	702	75	127	1,384	6·0
1829–30	640	55	904	113	156	1,868	6·6
1834–5	421	9	1,274	130	214	2,048	7·1
1839–40	465	48	1,044	227	168	1,952	12·0
1844–5	385	42	1,176	219	192	2,014	12·0
1849–50	331	66	1,216	180	179	1,972	9·6
1854–5	348	49	1,246	187	193	2,023	10·2

Table A3.3   Large provincial – Manchester Royal Infirmary* (cont.)

Year	Cured	Relieved	Other†	Dead	In house	Total	Mortality %
1859–60	191	74	1,554	255	181	2,255	12·3
1864–5	235	48	1,560	275	193	2,311	13·0
1869–70	213	122	1,725	306	186	2,552	12·9
1874–5	263	200	2,046	387	229	3,125	13·4

* Source: *Annual Reports.*

† This category includes, in addition to the usual reasons for dismissal, patients who were made out-patients or home-patients. These categories would indicate that either the patients did not need hospital treatment or were convalescing after a stay in hospital. It may also indicate severe pressure on bed space.

Table A3.4   Large provincial – Liverpool Royal Infirmary*

Year	Cured	Relieved	Other	Dead	In house	Total	Mortality %
1749–50	62	4	21	11	24	122	11·2
1749/50–							
1750/1	127	13	12	9	25	186	5·6
1755–6	135	23	41	15	46	260	7·0
1760–1	207	7	18	12	49	293	4·9
1765–6	301	8	18	14	62	403	4·1
1770–1	378	2	91	18	63	552	3·7
1775–6	277	22	35	17	65	416	4·8
1780–1	256	17	168	22	77	540	4·8
1785–6	377	36	274	25	84	796	3·5
1790–1	834	19	242	48	155	1,298	4·2
1795–6	741	35	194	34	142	1,146	3·4
1800	1,117	26	128	49	96	1,416	3·7
1805	724	39	111	32	102	1,008	3·5
1810	562	19	449	69	128	1,227	6·3
1815	565	70	451	53	136	1,275	4·7
1820	620	69	570	71	162	1,492	5·3
1825	755	80	633	70	198	1,736	4·6
1830	1,103	220	568	110	220	2,221	5·5
1835	1,194	357	171	121	206	2,049	6·6
1840	1,568	375	77	184	215	2,419	8·3

Table A3.4   Large provincial – Liverpool Royal Infirmary* (cont.)

Year	Cured	Relieved	Other†	Dead	In house	Total	Mortality %
1845	1,280	363	138	145	189	2,115	7·5
1850	1,428	421	268	139	187	2,443	6·2
1855	939	586	369	127	156	2,177	6·3
1860	1,104	661	197	180	177	2,319	8·4
1865	2,534	409	216	204	244	3,607	6·1
1870	1,553	671	170	178	220	2,792	6·9
1875	1,282	615	—	189	237	2,323	9·1

* Source: *Annual Reports.*
† This category includes patients who become out-patients.

Table A3.5   Scottish – Edinburgh Royal Infirmary*

Year	Cured	Relieved	Other	Dead	In house	Total	Mortality %
1755	257	79	76	14	60	486	3·3
1760	557	68	60	22	133	840	3·6
1765	528	56	87	41	120	832	6·7
1770	791	188	121	57	145	1,302	4·9
1775	1,523	101	93	61	184	1,962	3·4
1780	1,318	255	398	76	181	2,228	3·7
1785	1,274	170	196	103	164	1,907	5·9
1790	1,185	274	225	70	142	1,896	4·0
1795	1,062	143	269	95	167	1,736	7·0
1800	1,305	128	291	117	164	2,005	6·4
1805	1,504	122	214	83	180	2,103	4·3
1810	1,375	143	211	108	175	2,012	5·9
1815	1,065	168	300	111	145	1,789	6·0
1820	1,107	181	220	106	135	1,749	6·6
1825	1,953	260	194	274	220	2,901	9·6
1 Oct 1829– 1 Oct 1830	1,960	268	394	251	191	3,064	8·7
1 Oct 1834– 1 Oct 1835	2,345	555	249	251	215	3,615	7·4
1 Oct 1839– 1 Oct 1840	2,395	485	278	414	260	3,832	11·6

Table A3.5   Scottish – Edinburgh Royal Infirmary* (cont.)

Year	Cured	Relieved	Other	Dead	In house	Total	Mortality %
1 Oct 1844– 1 Oct 1845	2,047	578	284	369	257	3,535	11·3
1 Oct 1849– 1 Oct 1850	2,383	435	424	391	357	3,990	10·8
1 Oct 1854– 1 Oct 1855	2,212	906	453	392	434	4,397	9·9
1 Oct 1859– 1 Oct 1860	2,374	776	407	364	292	4,213	9·3
1 Oct 1864– 1 Oct 1865	2,731	867	443	492	366	4,899	10·9
1 Oct 1869– 1 Oct 1870	3,099	491	314	478	319	4,701	10·9
1 Oct 1874– 1 Oct 1875	2,374	1,292	510	430	404	5,010	9·3†

* Source: *Annual Reports.*
† Includes 71 deaths within 24 hours of admission – if these are excluded the mortality-rate falls to 7·3%.

Appendix 4 Summary of patients admitted to the Glasgow Royal Infirmary, 1800–70*

Year	Total	Medical	Surgical	Cured	Relieved	Dead	In house at end of year	No. of operations	Deaths after operations	Fever patients	Deaths fevers	Deaths medical	Deaths surgical	average no. of deaths	Average no. in house	Average length of stay (days)
1800	803	489	314	503	63	38	70	41								
1805	793	523	270	489	60	40	74	47								
1810	1,057	656	401	617	139	52	121	30								
1815	1,492	958	534	779	164	96	152	56								
1820	1,698	1,211	487	1,055	186	108	128	65								
1825	2,629	1,730	899	1,996	144	149	191	98								
1830	2,231	1,312	698	1,577	98	192	221	129								
1835	3,260	790	1,111	2,435	263	359	274	150		1,359	144	117	98			
1840	5,815	1,254	1,176	4,718	252	691	316	120		3,402	448	138	105	1:8·4	322	28
1845	2,993	1,075	1,383	2,144	317	234	207	175	22	535	75	148	86	1:9·68	234	25
1851	4,053	958	1,135	3,028	311	473	372	231	22	1,960	274	128	71	1:8·5	311	32
1855	3,416	1,153	1,397	2,217	556	360	333	199	18	866	128	157	75	1:9	271	28
1860	3,742	1,527	1,612	2,166	821	342	307	228	18	603	87	149	106	M1:10·7 F1:10·9	281	26½
1865	7,051	1,959	2,472	4,005	935	740	361	310	39	2,720	386	206	148	M1:8·03 F1:9·13	454	25½
1870	6,247	1,971	2,334	4,403	780	556	526	470	32	1,942	184	244	128	M1:10·24 F1:13·41	513· 34	28

Note: M = Males; F = Females. * Source: *Annual Reports* as shown. The figures are as first printed though discrepancies exist for some years. For 1800–30, the total does include patients who were dismissed or left voluntarily; for 1835–70, the total of those receiving treatment is greater than the figure for those admitted. Possibly patients in the house at the beginning and end of each year were excluded from this total.

Appendix 5   Cases admitted to the Newcastle and Manchester Infirmaries in the 1750s

Table A5.1   *Cases admitted to the Newcastle Infirmary from 23 May 1751 to 2 April 1752 inclusive**

	Admitted	Cured	Relieved	Other	Dead	In house at end of year
Abscesses and tumours	5		2	1	2	
Abscesses and tumours by amputation	3	3				
Agues	2	2				
Astma	3	1	1	1		
Cancer	2			1		1
Caries	1			1		
Caries by amputation	4				1	3
Catarrh						
Colic	1					1
Complication	5	1		4		
Consumption	10	1	2	6	1	
Contusions	3	2				1
Convulsions	1					1
Dislocations	2	2				
Dropsies	6	1		3	2	
Eyes disordered	7	3	1	2		1
Falling sickness	2	1		1		
Fever						
Fistula	3	1				2
Fluor albus	1	1				
Flux and bloody flux	6	3		3		
Fractures	8	5			1	2
Hysteric	1					
Inflammations	2	2				
Itch						
Mortification	1					1
Obstructions	7	2		5		

160

Table A5.1   Cases admitted to the Newcastle Infirmary from 23 May 1751 to 2 April 1752 inclusive* (cont.)

	Admitted	Cured	Relieved	Other	Dead	In house at end of year
Palsy	8	1	3			4
Piles						
Polypus	1	1				
Rheumatism, Sciatica, etc.	11	3	3	2		3
Ruptures	2		1	1		
Scalded	2	2				
Scald Head						
Scurvy	3	1		1	1	
Stone and Gravel	5	1	1	2		1
Strains	1	1				
Strumous, scrophulous, etc.	16		5	6		5
Strumous, scrophulous, etc. by amputation	6	3			2	1
Vertigo	1					1
Ulcers	17	10	1	1	1	4
Ulcers by amputation	1	1				
Weakness extreme	1	1				
Wens, etc.						
Wens, etc. by amputation	1	1				
Worms, etc.	1	1				
Wounds	4	2		2		1
Total	167	60	20	43	11	33

* Source: Newcastle Infirmary, *Annual Report*, 23 May 1751–2 April 1752.
The mortality-rate for the first year of the Newcastle Infirmary was 8·2 per cent.

Table A5.2   Cases admitted to the Manchester Infirmary from 24 June 1752 to 24 June 1754 inclusive*

	Admitted	Cured	Relieved	Dead	In house at end of year
Abscesses and tumours	122	75	10	7	30
Ague	2	2			
Astma	31	12	10		9
Burns and scalds	12	12			

Table A5.2   Cases admitted to the Manchester Infirmary from
24 June 1752 to 24 June 1754 inclusive* (cont.)

	Admitted	Cured	Relieved	Dead	In house at end of year
Cancer	2	1			1
Caries	23	15	2		6
Catarrh and coughs	16	8	2		6
Cholick and other pains	33	20	7	2	4
Complication	22	15	3	1	3
Contusions	9	9			
Consumption	24	5	6	2	11
Convulsions	9	3	2	1	3
Diabetes	1	1			
Dislocations and fractures	9	7			2
Dropsy	20	7	6	2	5
Erysiphelas	3	3			
Eyes disordered	51	36	6		9
Falling sickness	6	4	1		1
Fistula	3	3			
Flux and Bloody Flux	20	14	2	1	3
Hysterick and Hectick	28	16	8		4
Inflammations	14	12			2
Jaundice	1	1			
Leprosy and eruptions	32	26			6
Mortification	6	4		2	
Obstructions	19	12	2		5
Palsy	13	5	1		7
Pleurisy	1	1			
Piles	3	2	1		
Rheumatism	29	23	4		2
Ruptures	13	9			4
Scurvy	13	10	1		2
Scrophulous	58	23	12	4	19
Stone and gravel	11	9	1	1	
Surfeit	28	18	4		6
St Vitus's Dance	1	1			
Ulcers and other sores	129	90	7	2	30
Weakness and Lameness	33	20	5		8
Worms and Rickets	20	15			5
Uterine Disorders	12	8	1		3
Vomiting	1	1			
Lousy Evil	1	1			
Total	884	559	104	25	196

* Source: Manchester Infirmary, *Annual Report*, 24 June 1752–24 June 1754.
The mortality-rate for the first two years of the Manchester Infirmary was
3·6 per cent.

Appendix 6   A comparison of the mortality-rates presented by Florence Nightingale and Fleetwood Buckle

Table A6.1   F. Nightingale, Notes on Hospitals, *London, 1863*

	No. of special inmates on 8 April 1861	Average no. of inmates in each hospital	No. of deaths registered in 1861	Mortality on inmates %
In 106 principal hospitals of England	12,709	120	7,227	56·87
24 London hospitals	4,214	176	3,828	90·84
12 hospitals in large towns	1,870	156	1,555	83·16
25 county and important provincial hospitals	2,248	90	886	39·41
30 other hospitals	1,136	38	457	40·23
13 naval and military hospitals	3,000	231	470	15·67
1 Royal Sea Bathing Infirmary (Margate)	133	133	17	12·78
1 Dane Hill Metropolitan Infirmary (Margate)	108	108	14	12·96

The figures were taken from the *24th Annual Report of the Registrar-General* (1863) which contained a note stating that: 'The statement of the mortality of any One Hospital is qualified by the fact that the mortality is not deduced from the division of the deaths by the average number of patients, but by the number on one particular day' (p. 205). This note was not included in the table published by Miss Nightingale, thus creating a totally erroneous impression about the rate of mortality in hospitals.

Table A6.2   F. Buckle, Vital and Economical Statistics of the Hospitals, Infirmaries Etc. of England and Wales for the Year 1863, *London, 1865*

	No. of in-patients	No. of beds	Average no. of days in-patient on books	Total no. of deaths	Rate of mortality
117 hospitals of England and Wales	95,661	11,332	32·32	7,361	7·607
110 hospitals of England	94,712	11,168	32·25	7,334	8·202
7 hospitals of Wales	949	164	44·33 (Bangor)	27	3·58
18 metropolitan hospitals	35,031	3,738	32·17	2,856	9·19
92 English provincial hospitals	59,861	7,430	34·42	4,478	7·672

In this table the rate of mortality is calculated on the total number of in-patients in the year 1863, while in the table produced by Miss Nightingale it is calculated on the number of in-patients present on one day of the year, namely, 8 April 1861. The contrast in the rates of mortality thus calculated can be seen clearly. However, it was to be Miss Nightingale's figures which were to receive the greatest publicity despite the errors which were so plainly evident.

Appendix 7 Surgical operations, 1863[*]

Operations	Total no. of cases	Cured and relieved	Died	Rate of mortality %
Total no. of operations	3,440	3,150	290	8·43
Operations about eyes	1,122	1,122		
Total number (excluding eye operations)	2,318	2,028	290	12·51
Amputations	567	482	85	14·99
Hernia	169	125	44	26·03
Ovariotomy	22	5	17	77·27
Tumours, various	354	333	21	5·93
Tumours of breast, removed	70	60	10	14·28
Aneurism	7	5	2	28·57
Deligation of arteries	57	48	9	15·79
Paracentesis of abdomen, thorax and bladder	38	26	12	31·58
Lithotomy	80	70	10	12·5
Lithotrity	7	7	—	—

* Source: derived from the table prepared by Fleetwood Buckle in his survey of 117 hospitals in England and Wales, op. cit., Table II, p. 64.

Appendix 8   Deaths from pyaemia

Table A8.1   *Deaths from pyaemia compared to deaths from all causes in London hospitals**

Hospital	Time years	Total deaths	Deaths from pyaemia
Charing Cross	4	327	6
Guy's	2	954	7
St George's	1	319	7
London	1	318	13
St Mary's	2	341	5
St Thomas's	2	423	7
University	1	159	5
Royal Free	½	33	0
Total		2,874	50

* Source: J. S. Bristowe and T. Holmes, *The Hospitals of the United Kingdom*, p. 553.

Table A8.2   *Return of deaths from pyaemia in eight London hospitals**

Hospital	1869	1870	1871	1872	1873	1874	1875
St Bartholomew's	10	9	10	8	4	8	9
St George's	11	15	11	7	11	8	8
Guy's	21	23	28	19	29	30	38
London	10	7	17	22	19	29	27
Middlesex	4	6	10	7	8	9	3
Seamen's	4	5	9	8	5	10	7
St Thomas's	4	4	7	19	16	13	16
University	n.a.	n.a.	12	8	7	18	11
Total	64	69	104	98	99	125	119

* Source: derived from *9th Annual Report, Local Government Board*, 1879–80; appendix B, No. 3, p. 208.
Note: these figures for pyaemia should be related to the total number of patients who died in the hospitals. For example, in 1875, St Bartholomew's Hospital admitted 2,333 medical patients of whom 396 died and 3,705 surgical patients of whom 177 died. Therefore, the patients who died from pyaemia represented a very small percentage of the total deaths.

166

Notes

Chapter 1 Medical care and social policy

1 R. M. Clay, *The Medieval Hospitals of England*, xvii–xviii.
2 St Thomas's was not intended at first to be used as a hospital, but as an institution for the relief of the poor. The Letters Patent declared 'that the said late hospital in Southwark from henceforth may and shall be a place and home for poor persons there to be relieved and supported, and shall be called the House of the Poor in Southwark, in the county of Surry, near London of our foundation'.
3 Quoted in *Report of the Charity Commissioners – 1837*, p. 14.
4 St Bartholomew's Hospital, founded in 1123 and refounded in 1546; St Thomas's Hospital, founded in 1213 and refounded by Edward VI in 1551; St Mary's Bethlem, founded by Simon Fitzmary in 1247 as a convent, known to have been used for lunatics in 1403, refounded and handed over to the City in 1546; The Bridewell, founded in 1552 as a prison or reformatory; Christ's Hospital, founded in 1553 for fatherless and helpless children.
5 In addition to the chartered hospitals in London a smaller charity known as Bellott's Mineral Water Hospital was founded in 1610 at Bath. For wounded and disabled seamen the Greenwich Hospital was established.
6 Samuel Garth, *Oratoria Laudatoria*, p. 3.
7 Thomas De Laune, *Angliae Metropolis: or the present state of London*, p. 156.
8 By the provisions of his will the Observatory and Infirmary at Oxford were established.
9 Richard Mead certainly saw many patients without charging a fee.
10 C. Newman, *The Evolution of Medical Education in the Nineteenth Century*, p. 59.
11 Two quacks who received royal favour, William Read and John Taylor, were skilled oculists. Read trained as a jobbing tailor but left his trade to become an itinerant quack, travelling in the south of England. In 1684 he went to Dublin where he gained a reputation, and undoubtedly a skill, as an oculist and in couching cataracts. He then made his home in London where Queen Anne, who had weak eyes, appointed him as her oculist-in-ordinary, and in 1705 he was knighted for his free treatment of blinded soldiers and seamen and became well known in the literary circles of his time. Taylor was the son of a Norwich surgeon-apothecary and gained

practical experience in surgery as an apothecary's assistant in
London. He studied the surgery of the eye at St Thomas's and from
the age of twenty-four travelled over England for seven years. In
1736 he was appointed as oculist to George II and spent the
rest of his life operating on monarchs and writing books.

12 B. Abel-Smith, *The Hospitals 1800–1948*, p. 3.
13 Eliz., c. 2, 1601.
14 *London Post-Boy*, 14–16 April 1697.
15 Quoted in A. Rosenberg, 'The London Dispensary for the Sick-Poor', *Journal of the History of Medicine*, 14, 1959, p. 56.
16 Estimates as to the number of prescriptions given at the London Dispensary for the Sick-Poor vary according to the authorship of the figures. A proponent claimed in 1703 that approximately 20,000 prescriptions were written annually at a cost of a penny each. (R. Pitt, *The Craft and Frauds of Physick Expos'd*, p. 21.) A later and possibly more accurate estimate stated that: 'They began to make up Bills about the beginning of February 1697, and for the first Three Years, the number of Bills made up was thirteen thousand one hundred and ninety two, and in these last Three Years and ten Months (for the Calculation was taken December 1, 1704) they are increas'd to seventy one thousand nine hundred and ninety nine' (anon., *A Short Answer to a Late Book*, p. 34).

Chapter 2   To prove a need

1 'The origin and evolution of the 18th century hospital movement', *Hospital*, 17 January 1914, p. 429.
2 St Thomas More, 'The Best State of a Commonwealth and the New Island of Utopia', in E. Surtz, S.J., and J. H. Hexter (eds), *The Complete Works of St Thomas More*, vol. 4, pp. 139–41.
3 S. Hartlib, 'A Description of the Famous Kingdome of Macaria', 1641, in *Harleian Miscellany*, vol. 4, p. 382.
4 W. Petty, 'The Advice of W. P. to Mr. S. Hartlib for the Advancement of Some Particular Parts of Learning', in Marquis of Landsdowne (ed.), *The Petty Papers. Some unpublished writings of Sir William Petty*, vol. 1, pp. 263–76.
5 *England Wants: or several proposals probably beneficial for England*, pp. 4–8.
6 H. Chamberlen, *A Proposal for the Better Securing of Health. Humbly Offered to the Consideration of the Honourable House of Parliament*, pp. 1–2.
7 Petty, op. cit., vol. 2, p. 176.
8 Ibid.
9 N. Grew, 'The Meanes of a Most Ample Encrease of the Wealth and Strength of England in a Few Years Humbly represented to her Majestie In the Fifth Year of Her Reign', 1707, in E. A. Johnson, *Predecessors of Adam Smith: the growth of British economic thought*, pp. 117–28.
10 A. G. L. Ives, *British Hospitals*, p. 18.

11   'The origin and evolution of the 18th century hospital movement',
     Hospital, 17 January 1914, p. 429.
12   Ives, op. cit., p. 19.
13   Quoted in W. H. McMenemey, 'The hospital movement of the
     eighteenth century and its development', in F. N. L. Poynter (ed.),
     The Evolution of Hospitals in Britain, p. 47.
14   J. Bellers, *An Essay Towards The Improvement of Physick in
     Twelve Proposals*.
15   Ibid., p. 2.
16   Ibid.
17   Ibid., p. 3.
18   Ibid., p. 5.
19   Ibid., p. 6.
20   Ibid., pp. 7–9.
21   Quoted in 'The origin and evolution of the 18th century hospital
     movement', op. cit., p. 429.
22   Westminster Infirmary, *Annual Report*, 3 January 1721–2 to
     16 January 1722–3, 'An Account of the Proceedings of the Charitable
     Society for Relieving the Sick and Needy At The Infirmary in
     Petty-France, Westminster'.
23   These points will be considered in greater detail in subsequent chapters.
24   Quoted in 'The origin and evolution of the 18th century hospital
     movement', *Hospital*, 14 March 1914, p. 649.
25   Winchester County Hospital, *An Account of the Establishment of
     the County-Hospital at Winchester, with the Proceedings of the
     Governors, &c. from the first Institution on St. Luke's Day,
     October 18, 1736, to Michaelmas, 1737*; reprinted in Appendix 2.
26   *An Address to the Nobility, Gentry, Clergy and others, in behalf of a
     Public Infirmary erected at Liverpool*, 1 March 1748–9.
27   Quoted in 'The origin and evolution of the 18th century hospital
     movement', *Hospital*, 28 February 1914, p. 596.
28   Reprinted in 'An Account of the Rise and Establishment of the
     Infirmary, or Hospital for Sick-Poor, Erected at Edinburgh, 1730'.
29   *Monthly Chronicle*, 18 August 1729; quoted in A. Logan Turner,
     *Story of a Great Hospital: the Royal Infirmary of Edinburgh,
     1729–1929*, p. 50.
30   Eighteenth-century institutions for the infirm and the sick were
     usually called infirmaries if the community already possessed a
     charitable hospital for the aged. In some towns, especially those
     that acquired their voluntary hospital in the nineteenth century, the
     term 'infirmary' was reserved for the poor-law hospital and so was
     somewhat derogatory. (McMenemey, op. cit., p. 57.)
31   A list of the voluntary hospitals and the dates of their foundation
     is given in Appendix 1.

Chapter 3   Philanthropy or social enhancement

1   He was elected Dean of Exeter in 1741 and within nine months was
    calling for an infirmary of 160 beds.

2 The sermon was printed and dedicated to the Earl of Halifax, the first chairman of the committee appointed to run the county hospital.

3 R. Grey, D.D., *The Encouragement to Works of Charity and Mercy, from Christ's Acceptance of them as done to Himself*, p. 2.

4 D. Owen, *English Philanthropy 1660–1960*, p. 41.

5 Details of this scheme will be given in the final section of this chapter.

6 This privilege does not appear to have been an over-popular one as there were many instances of House Visitors not performing their duties: 'One of the Trustees is appointed weekly to visit the House, to enquire into the behaviour and conduct of the Patients, and to report his observations to the Weekly Board. But it is to be regretted that this service, so necessary to the good order of the House, is frequently neglected' (Hull General Infirmary, *Annual Report*, 1800).

7 'The Subscriptions would be totally inadequate to the Expense, did not the Charity receive additional Assistance from Collections, Legacies, and other Donations. . . . The Subscriptions fall so far short of the Expenditure, that the Charity could not subsist in its present Extent, if it did not receive about Nine Hundred Pounds per Annum of casual Benefactions' (General Infirmary at Leeds, *Annual Report*, 29 September 1796–29 September 1797).

8 J. M. Hall and V. C. Harral, *The General Hospital, Birmingham*, p. 1.

9 General Infirmary at Leeds, *Annual Report*, 29 September 1793–29 September 1794.

10 Hull General Infirmary, *Annual Report*, 1 January 1833–1 January 1834.

11 Select Committee on Metropolitan Hospitals 1890–93, *Third Report*, p. xcvii.

12 J. Duncumb, *A Sermon preached in the cathedral church of Hereford on Thursday, the third of August, 1797, at the annual meeting of the subscribers to the General Infirmary in that city*, p. 15.

13 *Directors and Prayers for the use of the Patients in the Hospital in Southwark; founded at the Sole Cost and Charges of Thomas Guy, Esq.*, p. 6.

14 J. Stonhouse, M.D., *Friendly Advice To a Patient To which are added Spiritual Directions For the Uninstructed*, p. 15.

15 W. H. McMenemey, 'The hospital movement of the eighteenth century and its development', in F. N. L. Poynter (ed.), *The Evolution of Hospitals in Britain*, p. 58.

16 Salisbury General Hospital, *Salisbury 200 – The Bi-centenary of Salisbury Infirmary, 1766–1966*, pp. 17–18.

17 York County Hospital, *An Account of the Publick Hospital for Diseased Poor in the County of York*, 1743, Order I. This was a typical ruling, though the monetary figures were often expressed in guineas.

18 An explanation of the position of Managers is given on p. 39.

19 A. Highmore, *Pietas Londiniensis*, London, 1810, p. 20.

Chapter 4 Hospital staff

1 Richard Mead, for example, was Physician to St Thomas's from 1703 to 1715.
2 York County Hospital, *An Account of the Publick Hospital for Diseased Poor in the County of York*, 1743, Order I.
3 *The Life of Sir Robert Christison Bart*, ed. by his sons, pp. 189–90.
4 Quoted in S. T. Anning, *The General Infirmary at Leeds: the first hundred years, 1767–1869*, vol. 1, p. 34.
5 'An Enquiry into the Present State of Polite Learning', in *The Works of Oliver Goldsmith*, vol. 2, pp. 64–5.
6 Radcliffe Infirmary, Oxford, *Minutes of the Board of Governors*, 21 July 1770.
7 W. H. McMenemey, 'The hospital movement of the eighteenth century and its development', in F. N. L. Poynter (ed.), *The Evolution of Hospitals in Britain*, pp. 64–5.
8 Quoted in W. Brockbank, *Portrait of a Hospital 1752–1948*, p. 35.
9 Ibid., p. 36.
10 These schools are mentioned in the proposal from the Manchester Infirmary: 'that persons destined to any branch of the medical profession, who have not had access to the most celebrated schools, should have the opportunity of acquiring the requisite qualification . . . without incurring an expense, which has hitherto operated not only as a discouragement but even as an exclusion' (ibid., pp. 35–6).
11 R. Stevens, *Medical Practice in Modern England*, pp. 11–12.
12 Royal College of Surgeons of Edinburgh in 1778; Royal College of Surgeons of Ireland in 1784; Royal College of Surgeons of London (later England) in 1800.
13 *Rules and Orders of the General Infirmary at Leeds*, 1767.
14 J. W. Willcock, *The Laws Relating to the Medical Profession*, pp. 30–1.
15 Ibid., pp. 56–7.
16 Ibid., p. 67.
17 *Rules and Orders of the Public Infirmary at Manchester*, 1752, Rules 55, 57, 58.
18 Quoted in Anning, op. cit., p. 48.
19 *Rules and Orders of the General Infirmary at Leeds*, 1767.
20 Quoted in Salisbury General Hospital, *Salisbury 200 – The Bi-centenary of Salisbury Infirmary, 1766–1966*, p. 13.
21 Quoted in Anning, op. cit., pp. 60–1.
22 T. Fuller, 'Exanthematologia (A Rational Account of Eruptive Fevers)', 1730, quoted in L. R. Seymer, *A General History of Nursing*, p. 63.
23 The author was writing about smallpox.
24 *Rules and Orders of the Public Infirmary at Manchester*, 1752, Rules 69, 70, 71.
25 F. Nightingale, 'Suggestions on the subject of providing, training and organizing nurses for the sick poor in workhouse infirmaries'

(letter to Sir Thomas Watson Bart, member of the committee appointed by the President of the Poor Law Board, London, 19 January 1867, p. 1), quoted in B. Abel-Smith, *A History of the Nursing Profession*, p. 5.

26 S. Wilks and G. T. Bettany, *A Biographical History of Guy's Hospital*, p. 80.
27 Quoted in *Salisbury 200*, op. cit., p. 70.
28 Charles Dickens, *Martin Chuzzlewit*, preface.
29 Quoted in E. T. Cook, *Life of Florence Nightingale*, p. 20. (Sarah Gamp was described as being a monthly nurse.)
30 *The Times*, 15 April 1857.
31 *Salisbury 200*, op. cit., p. 72.
32 The institutions referred to came into existence before Florence Nightingale began to influence the education and training of nurses.
33 Liverpool Royal Infirmary, *Annual Report*, 1855.
34 *The Lancet Commission on Nursing – Final Report*, p. 20.
35 Quoted in ibid., pp. 21–2.
36 Cf. T. Fuller, writing in 1730, on the ideal requirements for a nurse (see pp. 30–1).
37 'In 1887 the following hospitals, institutions, and organizations had matrons or superintendents who had been trained at the Nightingale School: the Westminster Hospital, St. Mary's Paddington, the Marylebone Infirmary, the Highgate Infirmary, the Metropolitan and National Nursing Association, the North London District Association, the Cumberland Infirmary, the Edinburgh Royal Infirmary, the Huntingdon County Hospital, the Leeds Infirmary, the Lincoln County Hospital, the Royal Infirmary, Liverpool, the Workhouse Infirmary, Liverpool, and the Southern Infirmary, Liverpool, the Royal Victoria Hospital at Netley, the Royal Hospital for Incurables, Putney, and the Salisbury Infirmary' (C. Woodham-Smith, *Florence Nightingale*, p. 567).
38 Fees for training nurses become a noticeable part of hospitals' income.
39 Abel-Smith, op. cit., pp. 34–5. Though the new nurses were generally superior to the old, not all were perfect as a case at Guy's Hospital in 1878 showed: 'Maria Grant, a nurse probationer from Job Ward, absconded from the Hospital on Thursday last with money to the account of 27 shillings belonging to 3 of the patients. She was apprehended on Monday and was found to have pawned one of the Hospital dresses which has been ordered by the magistrate to be delivered up' (diary of J. S. Steele, Superintendent, Guy's Hospital, reprinted as 'The Steele Diaries', 22 May 1878, no. III – Nurses, *Guy's Hospital Gazette*, 1949, 98–9).

Chapter 5 Admissions policy

1 R. Pinker, *English Hospital Statistics 1861–1938*, p. 57.
2 The first voluntary hospital opened in Wales was at Denbigh in 1807.

3   B. Abel-Smith, *The Hospitals 1800–1948*, p. 1.
4   J. K. Walker, 'Statistical observations on the medical charities of England and Ireland', *Transactions of the Provincial Medical and Surgical Association*, 4, 1836, 451.
5   Pinker, op. cit., derived from pp. 73, 81. The total of beds in all types of voluntary hospitals was 14,772.
6   B. R. Mitchell and P. Deane, *Abstract of British Historical Statistics*, Population and Vital Statistics, Table 2, p. 6.
7   Pinker, op. cit., p. 69.
8   *An Account of the Occasion and Manner of Erecting a Hospital at Lanesborough House near Hyde Park Corner – 8 February 1734.*
9   J. C. Lettsom, *Medical Memoirs of the General Dispensary in London*, p. 10.
10 J. Ferriar, *Medical Histories and Reflections*, vol. 1, p. 172.
11 Hull General Infirmary, *Annual Report*, 1827.
12 Hull General Infirmary, *Annual Report*, 1833.
13 Liverpool Infirmary, *Annual Report*, 5 March 1749/50–4 March 1750/51. Liverpool Infirmary, *Annual Report*, 4 March 1757–3 March 1758.
14 General Infirmary at Leeds, *Annual Report*, 27 September 1784–27 September 1785.
15 'An Account of the Rise and Establishment of the Infirmary, or Hospital for Sick-Poor, Erected at Edinburgh, 1730', p. 18.
16 Ibid.
17 Dumfries and Galloway Infirmary, *Annual Report*, 30 April 1784–30 April 1785. The figures for this year were:

From town and county of Dumfries	84
From Galloway	46
Soldiers	12
	142

18 The Salop Infirmary in its opening proposal stated that it would be 'for the Poor-sick and Lame of this County and Neighbourhood' (21 July 1737). This practice was condemned by a supporter of the Salisbury General Infirmary who wrote that as Salisbury was at the centre of good means of communication 'patients may at small expense be conveyed from considerable distances; as for instance, from Poole, Dorchester, Blandford, Devizes, Warminster, Lymington and Southampton, &c., &c. – A striking proof of the propriety of such an establishment at Salisbury, and of the absurdity of restricting a charity of this nature to any particular county' (*To the Printer of the* 'Salisbury Journal', *Blandford, 19 September 1766, by Your constant reader, A.Z.*). The open nature of the admission procedure at Sheffield General Infirmary was made explicit in the rules: 'That sick and lame Paupers of all Countries and Denominations be entitled to Admission to this Infirmary' (*Statutes and Rules*, 1813, Rule 40). In Scotland there were no rules restricting admission to hospitals, for example the Royal Northern Infirmary at Inverness served a very large area, as the

nearest infirmary to it was to the south at Aberdeen. The Infirmary accepted patients from all the northern counties with their widely-scattered communities.

19   *Regulations of the Infirmary of Aberdeen*, 1824. 'By the Charter of the Infirmary, the following are appointed Managers, viz:— The Provost, four Baillies, Dean of Guild, and Treasurer, the Provost of the preceding year, the Town Clerk, and the Convener of the Trades for the City of Aberdeen, all for the time; the Professor of Medicine in the Marischal College of Aberdeen; the Moderator of the Synod of Aberdeen for the time; and also every person who shall contribute and pay in the sum of £50 sterling or more; or who shall have subscribed, and who shall continue to pay £5 sterling or upwards yearly, for the use of the said Infirmary, in one payment, not less than the sum of £100 sterling. In addition to those before mentioned, Fourteen Managers are directed to be elected annually, at the general meeting on the first Monday of December; six of whom, at least, shall be chosen and taken from the following professions and societies within the city, viz:— One of the Ministers of Aberdeen, of the Established Church; one of the Managers of the Monies collected for pious uses at St. Paul's Chapel in the City of Aberdeen; two of the Physicians residing in Aberdeen; one of the Society of Shipmasters there; and one of the present or preceding Deacons of any of the Incorporate Trades within the said city; and that Four, at least, of the said Fourteen Managers shall, at every annual election, be charged and removed' (*Regulations of the Infirmary of Aberdeen*, 1838, frontispiece).

20   *The Orders and Constitutions of the Governors of the County Hospital, for Sick and Lame &c. at Winchester*, 18 October 1736.

21   Leicester General Infirmary, *Annual Report*, Midsummer 1773– Midsummer 1774.

22   Addenbrooke's Hospital, *Minute Book*, 4 August 1766.

23   *Rules and Orders of the Public Hospital in the Town of Cambridge*, 1778, Rule 66.

24   Bristol Infirmary, *Minute Book*, 3 September 1742.

25   Bristol Infirmary, *Minute Book*, 5 December 1797.

26   Radcliffe Infirmary, Oxford, *Rules and Orders*, 1798. A case occurred at the Northampton General Hospital where it was ordered that: 'Ann Lavender sent back being Lousy and to be admitted as soon as she is sent again if clean and wholesome' (*Minute Book*, 19 May 1753).

27   Quoted in K. J. Lowson and R. Grieve, *The Story of the Hull Royal Infirmary 1782–1948*, p. 7.

28   Hull General Infirmary, *Rules and Orders*, 1850, Rule 93.

29   Bristol Infirmary, *Minute Book*, 28 February 1739.

30   Sheffield General Infirmary, *General Quarterly Board Minutes*, 22 September 1800.

31   W. H. McMenemey, 'The hospital movement of the eighteenth century and its development', in F. N. L. Poynter (ed.), *The Evolution of Hospitals in Britain*, p. 56.

32   *A Report of the State of the General Hospital, near Birmingham,*
      29 September 1779.
33   *The Orders and Constitutions of the Governors of the County*
      Hospital, for Sick and Lame &c. at Winchester, 18 October 1736.
34   Winchester County Hospital, *Annual Report,* 25 June 1828–24 June
      1829.
35   General Infirmary at Leeds, *Quarterly Minute Book,* 23 March
      1770.
36   Ibid., 28 June 1780.
37   Hull General Infirmary, *Rules and Orders,* 1850, Rule 80.
38   Edinburgh Royal Infirmary, *Annual Report,* 1821.
39   Radcliffe Infirmary, Oxford, *Rules and Orders,* 1798.
40   *The Statutes of the Royal Infirmary of Edinburgh,* 1778, p. 76. 'Very
      early in the history of the Infirmary the grim spectre of the
      "waiting list" made its appearance. While cases of acute illness or
      of persons who had met with serious accidents were, in all
      circumstances, given first consideration there were numerous
      occasions when applications for the admission of those suffering
      from minor disabilities exceeded the available accommodation, and
      arrangements had to be made to cope with this difficulty. In the
      Statutes of the Infirmary, revised after the Charter had been
      granted, it was expressly stated that a sick person might be admitted
      as a "supernumerary" patient on the payment of sixpence per day
      till a bed on the ordinary establishment became vacant, this sum
      being considered sufficient for maintenance. As security one
      guinea had to be deposited with the Clerk of the House and when
      "the Depositum is consumed a new one is to be made; and, if
      there is any Remainder of any of them, it shall be returned at such
      Patients' going out." In some instances the supernumerary patients
      were cured so that their transference later to the wards occupied by
      the ordinary patients was unnecessary. In 1767, the managers
      accepted a proposal of the Earl of Galloway to lodge £5 sterling
      with the Clerk for the same purpose. When this sum became
      exhausted he promised to pay sixpence a day for any super-
      numerary patient who, in the opinion of the physicians, ought to be
      admitted to the house till vacant beds were available in the wards.
         'For a number of years a special return of this group of in-
      patients was made in the annual reports. In one year as many as
      eighty-seven were stated to have been under treatment. In 1771, the
      managers required that a monthly report should be made along
      with a statement of the names of those recommending their
      admission and of the number who had paid. On one occasion
      fifty-three supernumeraries were returned of whom only five had
      paid! This request for monthly returns suggested that some doubt
      had arisen as to the regularity with which the payments were being
      made. An arrangement existed, however, which gave the physicians
      discretionary power to admit supernumerary patients without
      payment, up to the number of ten, "who, from the nature of their
      ailment and poverty together, could not be rejected without doing

violence to the laws of humanity" ' (A. Logan Turner, *Story of a Great Hospital: The Royal Infirmary of Edinburgh, 1729–1929*, pp. 100–1).

41   General Infirmary at Leeds, *Annual Report*, 29 September 1774–29 September 1775.
42   *Rules and Orders of the Public Infirmary at Manchester*, 1752, Rule 44.
43   H. Bevan, *Records of the Salop Infirmary*, Table 8.
44   Sheffield General Infirmary, *Annual Report*, Midsummer 1854–Midsummer 1855.
45   J. K. Walker, M.D., *Observations on the Expediency of Establishing Hospitals*, p. 8.
46   P. Gaskell, *Artisans and Machinery – the moral and physical condition of the manufacturing population considered with reference to mechanical substitutes for human labour*, p. 206.
47   Quoted in F. F. Waddy, 'The early history of Northampton General Hospital', *Northampton General Hospital Clinical Reports* (reprint), 1964, p. 7.
48   London Hospital, *Initial appeal*, 1740.

Chapter 6   On the books

1   General Infirmary at Leeds, *Rules and Orders*, 1771, Rule 44.
2   Quoted in F. F. Waddy, 'The early history of Northampton General Hospital', *Northampton General Hospital Clinical Reports* (reprint), 1964, p. 5.
3   However, there is the problem of diagnosing an infectious case to be considered when discussing this point.
4   Quoted in A. E. Clark-Kennedy, *The London – A Study in the Voluntary Hospital System*, vol. 1, p. 27.
5   Manchester Infirmary, *Annual Report*, 25 June 1795–24 June 1796.
6   Dumfries and Galloway Royal Infirmary, *Annual Report*, Year ending 30 April 1789.
7   Liverpool Infirmary, *Annual Report*, 25 March 1748/9–5 March 1749/50.
8   Dumfries and Galloway Royal Infirmary, *Annual Report*, Year ending 11 November 1822.
9   Sheffield General Infirmary, *Annual Report*, Midsummer 1815–Midsummer 1816.
10   Manchester Infirmary, *Annual Report*, 24 June 1753–24 June 1754.
11   Birmingham General Hospital, *Annual Report*, Midsummer 1780–Midsummer 1781.
12   Birmingham General Hospital, *Annual Report*, Midsummer 1782–Midsummer 1783.
13   Salisbury General Infirmary, *Annual Report*, 31 August 1829–31 August 1830 (Report of the General Court held in February 1828).
14   Quoted in J. Langdon-Davies, *Westminster Hospital, 1719–1948*, p. 58.

15 Ibid.
16 General Infirmary at Leeds, *Annual Report*, 27 September 1774–29 September 1775.
17 The Leicester Infirmary admitted venereal patients almost from its opening, but they were segregated and were the subject of stringent rules as to behaviour and visiting, and the loss of any right to a second admission for a further re-infection.
18 Birmingham General Hospital, *Annual Report*, Midsummer 1829–Midsummer 1830. Prior to this date they were excluded from any form of treatment by the rules.
19 Manchester Infirmary, *Annual Report*, 25 June 1798–24 June 1799.
20 A separate fever hospital was established in 1804.
21 Quoted in C. Haskins, *The History of Salisbury Infirmary*, p. 10.
22 Ibid., p. 12.
23 Practice regarding the admission policies of hospitals for cases of fever and infectious disease will be discussed in subsequent chapters.
24 J. Aikin, M.D., *Thoughts on Hospitals;* and anon., 'Observations relating to the medical practice of an hospital', in *Statutes of the Royal Infirmary of Edinburgh*, 1778.
25 Ibid., pp. 88–9.
26 Aikin, op. cit., p. 33.
27 Ibid., p. 34.
28 Ibid., p. 35.
29 Ibid., p. 37.
30 Ibid., p. 40.
31 Ibid., p. 41.
32 Ibid., p. 42.
33 Ibid., p. 45.
34 Ibid., p. 51.
35 Ibid., p. 52.
36 *Oxford Journal*, 13 December 1777; quoted in A. G. Gibson, *The Radcliffe Infirmary*, pp. 200–1. The matron was dismissed as a result of this episode.
37 Northampton General Hospital, *Minutes*, 27 April 1771. No record is given of the birth.
38 Quoted in Clark-Kennedy, op. cit., p. 60.
39 Bristol Infirmary, *Rules and Orders*, 1742, Rule 6.
40 'Ordered that Thomas Cook, recommended by Mr. William Martin, having the Smallpox full on him and immediate Assistance necessary, be provided with a Lodging at hand and taken care of at the Expense of the Infirmary, and that Mr. Martin be acquainted that the Committee were surprised at his sending an Object so contrary to the rules of this Charity' (Clark-Kennedy, op. cit., p. 59).
41 Clark-Kennedy, op. cit., p. 60.
42 Winchester County Hospital, *Annual Report*, 6 July 1804–4 July 1805.
43 Glasgow Royal Infirmary, *Annual Report*, 1809.

44 E. Copeman, *Brief History of the Norfolk and Norwich Hospital*, p. 16.

45 Sheffield General Infirmary, *Annual Report*, Midsummer 1844– Midsummer 1845.

46 J. Clark, *A Collection of Papers, intended to promote An Institution for the Cure and Prevention of Infectious Fevers in Newcastle and other Populous Towns*, preface, pp. 38–9.

47 Ibid., p. 39.

48 The annual reports for the eighteenth century, giving information on the diseases treated and discharged, which are available and have been analysed for the purposes of this chapter have been obtained from the following institutions:

Aberdeen Royal Infirmary 1743, 1753–1815	Glasgow Royal Infirmary 1794–6
Devon and Exeter Hospital 1742–64	Manchester Infirmary 1752–4
	Newcastle Infirmary 1751–2
	St George's Hospital 1734–5
Dumfries and Galloway Royal Infirmary 1789	Westminster Hospital 1720–1
Edinburgh Royal Infirmary 1762–70	Worcester General Infirmary 1747
	York County Hospital 1740–3

Admission and discharge registers have been studied at the following hospitals:

Birmingham General Hospital	Devon and Exeter Hospital
	London Hospital
Bristol Infirmary	Newcastle Infirmary

49 Worcester General Infirmary, *Annual Report*, 18 October 1747– 14 October 1748. The less obvious diagnoses are: Empyema – matter in the chest (thorax); Albugo – white speck in the eye; St Vitus's Dance – erysipelas; Tinen – a mis-spelling for 'tinea', i.e. worms; Wound of the Selival Duet – wound of the salival duct.

50 This section is derived from G. C. Peachey, *History of St. George's Hospital*, pp. 198–200. Modern diagnoses for some of these complaints would be: Herpes – shingles; Chlorosis – 'green-sickness' – lack of menstrual discharge; Ophthalmis – inflammation of the eyes; Spina ventosa – 'caries' – a probably sarcomatous growth in the head of the tibia.

51 Langdon-Davies, op. cit., p. 28.

52 Westminster Hospital, *An Account of the Sick Poor January 3 1721/2 to January 16 1722/3 Inclusive*, pp. 6–10.

53 G. Munro-Smith, *A History of the Bristol Royal Infirmary*, p. 59. Again, some explanation of the diagnoses: Haemoptoe – haemoptysis – haemorrhage from the lungs; Painters' colic – lead poisoning; Leprosy – any common skin disease.

54 Bristol Infirmary, *Admissions Registers* for 1751, 1762 and 1779.

55 Quoted in J. Delpratt Harris, *The Royal Devon and Exeter Hospital*, p. 17.

56 Devon and Exeter Hospital, *Annual Reports*, 1742–6 to 1776–7. In the contemporary medical dictionaries 'Gutta Serena' is described as being 'dimness of sight'.

57 Manchester Infirmary, *Annual Report*, 24 June 1752–24 June 1754. *Abstract of Cases Admitted to the Infirmary for the Counties of Durham, Newcastle and Northumberland, 23 May 1751–2 April 1752;* reprinted in Appendix 5.

58 'An Account of the Rise and Establishment of the Infirmary, or Hospital for Sick-Poor, Erected at Edinburgh, 1730', in *Annual Report*, 6 August 1729–4 August 1730.

59 J. Patrick, *A Short History of Glasgow Royal Infirmary*, p. 17.

60 Quoted in T. C. Mackenzie (ed.), *The Royal Northern Infirmary, Inverness – The story of a Scottish Voluntary Hospital*, p. 20.

61 F. H. Jacob, *A History of the General Hospital near Nottingham*, pp. 64–7.

62 W. Shepherdson, *Reminiscences of the Hull General Infirmary*, p. 105.

63 The voluntary hospitals studied which have possessed such lists are:

Addenbrooke's Hospital, Cambridge 1836	Lincoln County Hospital 1835–6
	Manchester Infirmary 1838–9
Dumfries and Galloway Royal Infirmary 1822, 1835	Radcliffe Infirmary, Oxford 1837
Glasgow Royal Infirmary 1800, 1825, 1835	St George's Hospital 1829–30
	St Thomas's Hospital 1822
Gloucester Infirmary 1833–43, 1834–44, 1837	Sheffield General Infirmary 1798–1820

64 R. Ernest, *A Synopsis of Medical and Surgical Cases at the Sheffield General Infirmary During Twenty-Two Years*, p. 9.

65 Ibid., p. 9.

66 Ibid., pp. 2–8.

67 A Knight, 'On the grinders' asthma', *North of England Medical and Surgical Journal*, 1, 1830, 177.

68 Ibid.

69 Ibid.

70 P. Gaskell, *Artisans and Machinery – the moral and physical condition of the manufacturing population considered with reference to mechanical substitutes for human labour*, p. 206. The list of the diseases of the patients amplified the statement made by Gaskell quoted on p. 41.

71 Cf. 'a nervous spitting with paralytic tumours', 'atrophy with violent pains and eruptions' (quoted in Peachey, op. cit., p. 202) which were merely descriptions of the symptoms, while the later more accurate knowledgeable diagnoses were of paralysis and epilepsy.

72 A typical categorization was as follows (Liverpool Royal Infirmary, *Annual Report*, 1875):

(a) General Diseases

(b) Diseases of the Nervous System

(c) Diseases of the Circulatory System

(d) Diseases of the Absorbent System

(e) Diseases of the Respiratory System

(f) Diseases of the Digestive System

(g) Diseases of the Urinary System

(h) Diseases of the Generative System

(i) Diseases of the Female Breast

(j) Diseases of the Organs of Locomotion

(k) Diseases of the Skin and Cellular Tissue

(l) Poison

(m) Injuries

(n) Diseases not included in the above

73   J. S. Bristowe and T. Holmes, *The Hospitals of the United Kingdom, Sixth Report of the Medical Officer of the Privy Council*, 1863, appendix 15.

74   'In the light of history, it may be said that the most significant change which occurred in the voluntary hospitals in the first half of the nineteenth century was the growing emphasis on the acute sick. To a considerable extent, the trend marked the triumph of the "honorary doctors" over those of the charitable public. Many of the latter were content to have their money used to give relief and comfort to those in pain: help to a patient whose suffering was of long duration might even be preferred to constructive treatment for a patient whose stay was short. Pain was what mattered, not any "economic" return for money spent. The doctors on the other hand and those lay governors who were influenced by them wanted to show results in terms of cure, and they were naturally reluctant to surround themselves with cases which showed the limitations of their professional skill. Doctors who taught particularly wanted to demonstrate successes' (B. Abel-Smith, *The Hospitals 1800–1948*, pp. 44–5). This statement is in contrast with the arguments presented in this chapter, which would suggest that this change did not take place until the second half of the nineteenth century.

Chapter 7   Fever cases

1   See P. A. Richmond, 'Glossary of historical fever terminology', *Journal of the History of Medicine*, 16, 1961.

2   In general the physicians left the city with their patients and it was left to the apothecaries to treat the remaining population.

3   W. Blizard, *Suggestions for the Improvement of Hospitals and Other Charitable Institutions*, pp. 44–5. This comment will have considerable relevance when the evidence on 'hospital diseases' is examined.

4   J. Clark, *A Collection of Papers, intended to promote An Institution for the Cure and Prevention of Infectious Fevers in Newcastle and other Populous Towns, Report of the Committee*, p. 47.

5   Ibid., pp. 47–8.

6   This was the case at the Newcastle Infirmary where fevers of a low type were admitted under the pretence of 'rheumatism' or 'catarrh'. See p. 54.

7   J. Clark, op. cit., 'Postscript-letter to Dr. Clark, from Dr. Currie (of Liverpool), 24 August, 1802', pp. 237–8.

8   Ibid., p. 48.

9   J. Howard, *An Account of the Principal Lazarettos in Europe*, p. 208. A plan was put forward at the Norfolk and Norwich Hospital in 1780 to erect a separate building for the treatment of infectious disorders, but the scheme was abandoned as the Medical Officers reported against it.

10 Chester Infirmary, Rule 2, quoted in ibid., p. 209.

11 Quoted in W. Brockbank, *Portrait of a Hospital 1752–1948*, p. 28.

12 Quoted in ibid., p. 32. Cf. the Chester General Infirmary where fever patients were accepted from the town. At Manchester the plan was only to treat those who had contracted the fever in the Infirmary. The same principles of separation were to apply at both institutions.

13 J. Ferriar, *Medical Histories and Reflections*, vol. 3, p. 72.

14 Ibid., pp. 80–1.

15 T. Bernard, 'Extracts from a further account of the House of Recovery at Manchester', *The Reports of the Society for Bettering the Condition and Increasing the Comforts of the Poor*, vol. 2, p. 125.

16 John Clark when collecting his evidence for fever wards in New-castle collected the views of Dr Matthew Baillie, Dr Heberden, Dr Saunders, Dr Lettsom, Dr Willan, Dr Ferriar of Manchester, Dr Haygarth of Chester, Dr Falconer of Bath, Dr Beddoes of Bristol, Drs Gregory, Hamilton and Rutherford of Edinburgh, etc., who were agreed on the principle of separation.

17 A. Highmore, *Pietas Londiniensis: The History, Design and Present State of the Various Public Charities In and Near London*, p. 111. The above statement is not strictly true, as a hospital for the treatment of and inoculation against smallpox had been opened in January 1747. 'Every person destitute of friends or money, and labouring under this disease, was and is still deemed a proper object of the charity' (ibid., p. 278). The hospital made various moves until it settled in a new building at St Pancras in June 1794. Vaccination was introduced on 21 January 1799 and in the space of three years 9,000 were vaccinated 'and no complaint of any ill-success had then appeared; these were chiefly children under five years of age' (ibid., p. 296).

18 Hull General Infirmary, *Annual Report*, 1803.

19 Quoted in W. Shepherdson, *Reminiscences of the Hull General Infirmary*, p. 75.

20 T. H. Bickerton, *A Medical History of Liverpool from the Earliest Days to the Year 1920*, p. 33. There had been an abortive attempt in 1801 to set aside wards at the Middlesex Hospital for the use of the 'Institution for the Cure and Prevention of Contagious Fevers'.

21 Quoted in Salisbury General Hospital, *Salisbury 200 – The Bicentenary of Salisbury Infirmary, 1766–1966*, p. 21.

22 Radcliffe Infirmary, Oxford, *Special General Court*, 22 April 1818; quoted in A. G. Gibson, *The Radcliffe Infirmary*, p. 39.

23 Nottingham General Hospital, *Annual Report*, June 1827–June 1828.

N

24   'Any patient affected with continued, remittent, or scarlet fever, measles, small-pox, or other contagious disease, may be admitted on any day of the week, and without the recommendation of a Governor, by the Surgeon Apothecary, either on his personal inspection, or on the certificate of a regular medical practitioner, stating the particular disease, but notice must be given to the Surgeon Apothecary and his instructions followed respecting the time and manner of the patient being brought into the Hospital' (ibid.).

25   C. Haskins, *The History of Salisbury Infirmary*, p. 15.

26   Ibid., p. 19.

27   Shepherdson, op. cit., pp. 76–7.

28   Quoted in H. St G. Saunders, *The Middlesex Hospital 1745–1948*, p. 98.

29   Quoted in J. Langdon-Davies, *Westminster Hospital, 1719–1948*, p. 88.

30   Ibid. In 1854 it was claimed that of 165 cases of cholera admitted only 12 died.

31   Birmingham General Hospital, *Annual Report*, Midsummer 1829– Midsummer 1830.

32   Lincoln County Hospital, *Annual Report*, 24 June 1839–24 June 1840.

33   J. D. Leader and S. Snell, *Sheffield Royal Infirmary, 1797–1897*, p. 43.

34   This view should be judged in relation to the comments made in 'Observations relating to the medical practice of an hospital', in *Statutes of the Royal Infirmary of Edinburgh*, 1778; see pp. 49–50.

35   A. K. Chalmers, *The Health of Glasgow 1818–1925 – An Outline*, pp. 153–4.

36   Glasgow Royal Infirmary, *Annual Report*, 1817.

37   Patients suffering from 'continued fever' represented 714 out of the 1,886 patients treated during the year (1817).

38   A. Logan Turner, *Story of a Great Hospital: The Royal Infirmary of Edinburgh, 1729–1929*, p. 158.

39   Edinburgh Royal Infirmary, *Annual Report*, 1818.

40   'History of Aberdeen Royal Infirmary – its rise and progress', reprinted from *People's Journal*, 1904, p. 7.

41   Quoted in J. S. Riddell, *The Records of the Aberdeen Medico-Chirurgical Society from 1789 to 1922*, p. 29.

42   Ibid., p. 30.

43   Quoted in ibid., pp. 33–4.

44   Ibid., pp. 690–1.

45   J. S. Bristowe and T. Holmes, *The Hospitals of the United Kingdom*.

46   Ibid., p. 520.

47   Ibid. 1861 was the first year that the classification and separation of patients were undertaken at the London Fever Hospital.

48   'At Guy's Hospital there was a great outbreak of typhus towards the end of 1862; into one ward containing 50 patients 1 or 2 typhus cases were admitted, and the disease spread rapidly; no fewer than 7 patients in this ward took the fever, which in 5

instances was fatal' (C. Murchison, *A Treatise on the Continued Fevers of Great Britain*, p. 692).

49 Anon., 'On the necessity for separate wards for fever cases in general hospitals', *Lancet*, 11 February 1865; reprinted in *Half-Yearly Abstract of the Medical Sciences*, 41, January–June 1865, pp. 25–6.

50 Ibid., 26.

51 E. L. Fox, 'Where should typhus be treated?', *Edinburgh Medical Journal*, January 1866; reprinted in *Half-Yearly Abstract of the Medical Sciences*, 43, January–June 1866, pp. 2–3.

52 Bristowe and Holmes, op. cit., footnote on p. 470.

53 T. Jones, 'On the recent outbreak of small-pox at St. George's Hospital', *St. George's Hospital Reports*, 5, 1870, p. 233.

54 J. C. Steele, 'The mortality of hospitals, general and special, in the United Kingdom, in times past and present', *Journal of the Statistical Society*, 40, 1877, p. 203. This essay was awarded the Howard Prize Medal for 1876.

55 The provision of treatment for fever cases will be of importance when the methods of dealing with outbreaks of 'hospital diseases', which included typhus, are considered in chapter 9.

Chapter 8 Surgery

1 The governing authorities of the voluntary hospitals already allowed their surgeons to have apprentices who were able to walk the wards, though not to practise surgery.

2 The original regulations demanded that a candidate had to be at least twenty-five years of age and have a certificate of good character. It was necessary that he had spent six years in professional study, at least three in a recognized hospital and one acting as a house surgeon or surgical dresser in a recognized hospital in the United Kingdom. A further requirement for entry was the submission of a written account of at least six clinical cases. The examination, held in two parts with a day's interval between, was composed of written papers on anatomy and physiology, surgery, pathology and therapeutics. The papers were answered between ten and five each day and the candidate could be additionally questioned orally by the examiners, and could be required to perform dissections and operations on cadavers.

3 F. F. Cartwright, *The Development of Modern Surgery*, p. 4. For an example of the training received by surgeons, see V. Mary Crosse, *A Surgeon in the Early Nineteenth Century*. This is an account of the life of J. G. Crosse (1790–1850) who trained initially under a surgeon at Swaffham, Norfolk, and eventually at a number of the hospitals in London.

4 Note the activities of the 'Resurrectionists'.

5 The famous diarist Samuel Pepys underwent the ordeal of this operation and regularly celebrated on the anniversary of its performance its successful outcome.

N*

6   See pp. 78–9.
7   *Rules and Orders of the Public Infirmary at Manchester*, 1752, Rule 50. In 1765 this rule was amended by adding 'and that twenty-four hours previous notice be given of such consultation in writing by the Apothecary' (quoted in W. Brockbank, *Portrait of a Hospital*, p. 23).
8   There was an eighteenth-century word 'bottom' which meant that all discomforts and pains of life were to be borne cheerfully. Bottom was needed to bear the pain and shock of surgical treatment.
9   W. J. Bishop, *The Early History of Surgery*, p. 155.
10 Worcester General Infirmary, *Annual Report*, 18 October 1747–14 October 1748.
11 Glasgow Royal Infirmary, *Annual Report*, 8 December 1794–1 January 1796:

Trepan	2	Cancerous Eye	1
Amputation	8	Cancerous Lip	4
Hydrocele	3	Cancerous Nose	1
Aneurism	1	Cancerous Breast	2
Tapping	2	Extracting Gland from Axilla	1
Fistula in Ano	2	Imperforate Nostril	1
Fistula Lachrymalis	2	Extraction of Polypi from the ear	1
Double Hair Lip	1		—
			32

Glasgow Royal Infirmary, *Annual Report*, 31 December 1799–31 December 1800:

Amputations	5	Fistula in Ano	3
Stone	1	Extirpation of cancerous tumours	2
Cancerous Breasts	4	Tying Ulnar Artery	1
Cancerous Lips	5	Tying Vena Saphena	1
Hydrocele	10	Empyema	1
Couching	3	Tapping	2
Polypus	3		—
			41

12 J. P. Halton, *The Results of the Great Operations of Surgery During a Practice of Twenty-Two Years:*

Amputations of the thigh	1 death in 11
Amputations of the leg	1 death in 6
Amputations of the arm	1 death in 18
Amputations of the hand or foot	1 death in 36
Excision of Joints	1 death in 7
Lateral operations on the bladder	1 death in –
Ligatures on aneurisms	1 death in –
Strangulated bowel, Femoral Inguinal and Scrotal hernia	1 death in 4
Partial removal of bones for compound fractures – leg	4 deaths in 35
thigh	1 death in 4
humerus	1 death in 4

| | fore-arm and hand | 2 deaths in 7 |
| | Removal of tumours | 4 deaths in 25 |

(This table is compiled from figures given in the above text.)
Ligaturing of aneurisms consisted of the comparatively simple, yet very dangerous, procedure of tying the artery with a silk ligature to occlude it. This was done to bypass an aneurism, the weakening and ballooning of an arterial wall caused by injury or by untreated syphilis.

13 Liverpool Infirmary, *Annual Report*, 1836.

Operations performed from March 1834 to March 1836:

	Admitted	Cured	Died
Amputations of upper extremities, including one of the shoulder joint	20	19	1
Amputation of lower extremities – three individuals lost two legs each	23	21	2
	43	40	3
Tumours removed, including diseased mammae	10	8	2
Lithotomy – lateral operation	2	2	–
Operation for strangulated hernia	4	3	1
Reduced by the taxis (4) – operations of less importance, including tapping	21	18	3
	37	31	6
Total	80	71	9

The operation for hernia was an attempt at relief of an acutely obstructed bowel. Taxis was the method of pushing the bowel back through the constricting ring of the hernial sac into the abdominal cavity. If this failed an open operation had to be attempted.

14 The notebook giving details of the operations was lent by Dr Critchley to Dr S. T. Anning of Leeds, who has kindly allowed its use for this analysis.

15 Though speed was required in the performance of surgical operations the records of lithotomy operations by surgeons such as W. Cheselden who it was said could remove a stone in less than a minute did not include the time for staunching the flow of blood or the suturing of the wound.

16 Brockbank, op. cit., pp. 61–2.

The 110 operations were described as follows:

Amputation of the leg	40	Cataract	9
Amputation of the arm	22	Trepan	3
Hernia	8	Aneurysm	2
Tumours	8	Tracheotomy	2
Lithotomy	7	Hare-lip	1
Contracture after burns	6	Various	2

17   *Answers by the Managers of the Royal Infirmary of Edinburgh, to Questions transmitted to them by the Committee appointed by the House of Commons to inquire into the state of Medical Practice and Education*, 1834, p. 2.

Capital operations	1830–1	1831–2	1832–3	1833–4
Lithotomy	2	5	11	10
Lithotrity	0	0	0	1
Amputations	15	3	13	29
Excision of head of humerus	0	1	0	0
Excision of elbow-joint	0	0	1	4
Ligature of common iliac artery	1*	0	0	0
Ligature of external iliac	0	0	0	1
Ligature of femoral artery	4*	0	0	0
Ligature of brachial artery	0	0	1	1
Hernia	3	2	2	4
Tumours	2	0	2	0
Excision of mamma	1	4	2	7
Excision of testicle	0	0	1	3
Excision of upper jaw	2	0	1	0
Excision of lower jaw	0	0	1	1
Trapan	1	0	0	2
Tracheotomy	0	0	2	0
Extirpation of eye	0	0	1	0

Note: The cases of ligature of artery marked by asterisks were for checking secondary haemorrhage. The others were for aneurism.

18   Salisbury General Hospital, *Salisbury 200 – The Bi-centenary of Salisbury Infirmary, 1766–1966*, p. 27.
19   Cartwright, op. cit., pp. 24–5.
20   E. A. Underwood, 'Dumfries and the early history of surgical anaesthesia', *Annals of Science*, 23, 1967.
21   Cartwright, op. cit., p. 32.
22   F. F. Waddy, 'The early history of Northampton General Hospital', *Northampton General Hospital Clinical Reports* (reprint), 1964, p. 7.
23   *Medical Gazette*, 3 December 1847.
24   Newcastle Infirmary, *Annual Report*, 1 April 1849–31 March 1850.
25   W. M. Coates, *On Chloroform and Its Safe Administration*, pp. 23–4.
26   Ibid., p. 24.
27   Newcastle Infirmary, op. cit.
28   F. Buckle, *Vital and Economical Statistics of the Hospitals, Infirmaries Etc. of England and Wales for the Year 1863*, p. 64. The survey was made by means of a questionnaire which was completed by the hospitals themselves and is subject, therefore, to an unknown degree of error.
29   The other major factors involved (assuming equal skills between surgeons) being the types of cases operated upon and the sanitary conditions of the hospital. From the records of the hospitals it would appear that the operations performed at the different hospitals varied very little, irrespective of size or position. In any case, even the new operations such as ovariotomy were few in

number and would only marginally affect the overall surgical
mortality. Sanitary conditions will be examined in chapter 9.

30   Buckle, op. cit., p. 75.
31   Cartwright, op. cit., pp. 44–5.
32   This will be examined in chapter 9.
33   General Infirmary at Leeds, *Annual Report*, 1860.
34   General Infirmary at Leeds, *Annual Report*, 1875. This figure did
     not include the 381 eye and ear operations which were also carried
     out.
35   Quoted in H. Graham, *Surgeons All*, p. 363.
36   J. A. Lawrie, 'On the results of amputations', *London Medical
     Gazette*, 1 (new series), 1841, 394.
37   In this section on amputation only removal of limbs will be dealt
     with, thus excluding consideration of the removal of breasts.
38   J. Poland, *A Retrospect of Surgery during the Past Century*, p. 21.
     The figure quoted includes all types of surgical operations, major
     and minor, but as the bulk of surgery undertaken was that of
     amputation, it was amputation which influenced the death-rate
     more than any other operation.
39   Halton, op. cit., derived from pp. 15–17. For complete details, see
     p. 185. Amputation of the leg refers to below-knee amputation.
40   J. C. Steele, 'The mortality of hospitals, general and special in the
     United Kingdom, in times past and present', *Journal of the
     Statistical Society*, 40, 1877, 208.
41   Medical Society of Observation, *Statistical Reports of Amputations,
     Compound Fractures, Operations for Hernia and Lithotomy in
     London Hospitals*, Table of cases of amputations.
42   J. H. James, 'On the causes of mortality, after amputation of the
     limbs', *Transactions of the Provincial Medical and Surgical Associa-
     tion*, 18 (new series), 5, 1851, p. 52.
43   J. P. Potter, 'Results of amputations at University College Hospital,
     London, statistically arranged', *Medico-Chirurgical Transactions*,
     24, 1841, p. 156.
44   J. M. Chelius, *A System of Surgery*, trans. with additional notes by
     J. F. South, pp. 905–6. The quotation from the notes of J. F.
     South illustrates that until the introduction of anaesthesia in 1846
     shock was considered to be a prime cause of death. The problem
     posed by hospital diseases will be considered in chapter 9.
45   Steele, op. cit., p. 208.
46   E. L. Hussey, 'Statistical report of cases of amputation, lithotomy,
     and hernia, in the Radcliffe Infirmary, Oxford', *Transactions of the
     Provincial Medical and Surgical Association*, 7, 1853, p. 96.
47   Ibid., 98.
48   'Report of the committee on the uses and effects of chloroform',
     Medico-Chirurgical Transactions, 47, 1864, Appendix D, pp.
     428–31.
49   J. S. Bristowe and T. Holmes, *The Hospitals of the United Kingdom*,
     p. 559.
50   Buckle, op. cit., Table II, p. 64.

51 Dumfries and Galloway Royal Infirmary, *Annual Report*,
12 November 1864–11 November 1865, Medical and Surgical
Report.

52 T. Nunneley, *Operations Performed at the General Infirmary at
Leeds*, pp. 20–1.

53 *St. Bartholomew's Hospital Reports*, 12, 1876; derived from pp. 73–4.
These figures cover the introduction of antisepsis in 1865 which
will be discussed in chapter 9, where its impact on the mortality-
rate after amputation will be assessed.

54 Excision, the practice of removing only the diseased joint, did not
come into common usage until after the introduction of anaesthesia
because of the prolonged nature of the operation and the resultant
pain.

55 It has been suggested that this part of the Hippocratic Oath refers
to castration rather than lithotomy, though the evidence is not well
documented.

56 A. Miller, *An Inquiry into the Average Mortality in Lithotomy
Cases: with a few remarks on the operation of lithotrity*, pp. 6–7.

57 W. Cheselden, *The Anatomy of the Humane Body*, p. 334.

58 R. Smith, 'A statistical inquiry into the frequency of stone in the
bladder in Great Britain and Ireland', *Medico-Chirurgical Transactions*, 11, part 1, 1820, p. 20.

59 Ibid., pp. 39–40.

60 Ibid., p. 43.

61 Ibid., p. 43.

62 A. Marcet, *An Essay on the Chemical History and Medical Treatment of Calculous Disorders*, footnote on p. 29. The discrepancy in
the evidence presented for the Hereford General Hospital by
Smith and by Dobson cannot be accounted for as the relevant
information on in-patients is not available.

63 P. M. Martineau, 'On lithotomy', *Medico-Chirurgical Transactions*,
11, part 2, 1821, p. 412.

64 Marcet, op. cit., pp. 23–4.

65 Martineau, op. cit., p. 405.

66 J. Yelloly, *Remarks on the Tendency to Calculous Diseases*, p. 60.

67 Ibid., p. 62.

68 Steele, op. cit., p. 207.

69 Ibid.

70 Hussey, op. cit., p. 99.

71 Ibid., p. 100.

72 Medical Society of Observation, op. cit., Table of cases of operations for stone in the bladder at the London hospitals.

73 'Statistical analysis of 186 lithotomy operations', *Medical Times and
Gazette*, 18 (new series), 1859, p. 32.

74 T. Bryant, 'An analysis of 230 cases of lithotomy', *Medico-
Chirurgical Transactions*, 45, 1862, p. 330. The overall figure given
by the *Medical Times and Gazette* was 1 in 13·6, while the figure
given here was 1 in 21½.

75 Buckle, op. cit., p. 64.

76 A. Poland, 'Urinary calculi and lithotomy', in T. Holmes (ed.), *A System of Surgery*, vol. 4, p. 461.
77 Bristowe and Holmes, op. cit., p. 563.

	Total	Deaths	Mortality (%)
London hospitals	135	19	14·07
Large provincial towns	288	35	12·15
Small or rural towns	144	24	16·67

78 H. Coote, 'On lithotomy and lithotrity', *St. Bartholomew's Hospital Reports*, 4, 1868, p. 132.
79 Nunneley, op. cit., p. 10.
80 Miller, op. cit., p. 39.
81 'Statistical analysis of twenty-one lithotrity operations', *Medical Times and Gazette*, 18 (new series), 1859, p. 59.
82 C. Hawkins (ed.), *The Works of Sir Benjamin Brodie*, vol. 2, p. 679.
83 Nunneley, op. cit., p. 10.
84 Ibid., pp. 10–11.
85 Coote, op. cit., p. 140.
86 C. Hawkins, 'Lithotrity', in T. Holmes (ed.), *A System of Surgery*, Vol. 4, p. 490.
87 Cartwright, op. cit., pp. 180–1.
88 Ibid., pp. 181–2.
89 Steele, op. cit., p. 270.
90 Hussey, op. cit., p. 101.
91 Ibid., p. 102.
92 Medical Society of Observation, op. cit., Table of cases of strangulated hernia.
93 Buckle, op. cit., p. 64.
94 Bristowe and Holmes, op. cit., p. 558.
95 Nunneley, op. cit., p. 11.
96 Ibid., p. 12.

Chapter 9 Hospital diseases

1 R. Lawson Tait, *An Essay on Hospital Mortality*, pp. 3–4.
2 J. Pringle, *Observations on the Nature and Cure of Hospital and Jayl-Fevers*, pp. 4–5. The use of the word 'humours' should be noted.
3 Ibid., p. 8.
4 T. Brocklesby, *Oeconomical and Medical Observations in Two Parts from the year 1758 to the year 1763*, London, 1764, pp. 58–9.
5 J. Aikin, *Thoughts on Hospitals*, London, 1771.
6 W. Blizard, *Suggestions for the Improvement of Hospitals and Other Charitable Institutions*, pp. 35–6.
7 T. Sympson, *A Short Account of the Old and of the New Lincoln County Hospitals*, p. 5. The Lincoln County Hospital was first opened in 1777.
8 P. Clare, *An Essay on the Cure of Abscesses by Caustic, and on the Treatment of Wounds and Ulcers; with some observations on some improvements in surgery*, pp. 50–1.

9   Liverpool Infirmary, *Annual Report*, 4 March 1771–2 March 1772.
10 Liverpool Infirmary, *Annual Report*, 5 March 1781–4 March 1782.
11 T. Champney, *A Review of the Healing Art*, p. 100.
12 M. C. Buer, *Health, Wealth, and Population in the Early Days of the Industrial Revolution*, p. 134.
13 J. Howard, *An Account of the Principal Lazarettos in Europe*, 1789. It is worth while noting that although Howard visited and reported on all the London hospitals in existence at this time, he visited only twelve out of a possible twenty-five hospitals in the provinces.
14 Ibid., p. 141.
15 Ibid., p. 132.
16 Ibid., p. 134. The comments of Sir Gilbert Blane in 1813 about St Thomas's Hospital are worth noting in this context: 'There were formerly near 500 beds; but in the year 1783, when I was elected physician, febrile infection prevailed so much, that my two immediate predecessors, and one of the surgeons, besides several of the medical attendants, had died in the course of the preceding year of fever caught in the hospital, upon which the number of patients was reduced, and new methods of cleanliness and ventilation were adopted. From this date the wards were white-washed annually, hygiene was improved, and apertures were provided at the tops of windows. Iron bedsteads had been adopted before this time, as less likely to contract and retain infection than those made of wood. . . . In consequence of these precautions, no medical attendant has since been affected with the hospital fever; not could I ascribe more than three or four deaths of nurses and patients to this cause during the whole time of my incumbency' (G. Blane, 'On the comparative prevalence and mortality of different diseases in London', *Medico-Chirurgical Transactions*, 1, 1813, pp. 112–13).
17 Howard, op. cit., p. 135.
18 Ibid., p. 136.
19 Ibid., p. 154.
20 Ibid., p. 160.
21 Ibid., p. 173.
22 Ibid., p. 190.
23 Ibid., p. 192. It is interesting to note that in 1781 the Board of the General Infirmary at Leeds had ordered: 'That Mr. Hanson pursue the same Methods to prevent the Increase of Bugs as formerly practised' (quoted in S. T. Anning, *The General Infirmary at Leeds*, vol. 1, p. 13).
24 Howard, op. cit., p. 131.
25 Ibid., p. 171.
26 M. Wall, *A Letter to John Howard, Esq., F.R.S.*
27 J. Howard, *The State of the Prisons in England and Wales*, p. 199.
28 Quoted in W. Brockbank, *Portrait of a Hospital*, p. 24. Note, the third ruling authorized the practice of putting two patients in one bed if there was great pressure on the resources of the infirmary.

29 F. Renaud, *A Short History of the Rise and Progress of the Manchester Royal Infirmary from the Year 1752 to 1877*, p. 28. In the annual report for 1787–8 the improvements are mentioned, though the reasons for their implementation are not given. The fourth recommendation should be noted in the context of the strictures made by John Howard about the sanding of floors.

30 J. Clark, *A Collection of Papers, intended to promote An Institution for the Cure and Prevention of Infectious Fevers in Newcastle and other Populous Towns*, supplement, p. 215.

31 Ibid., pp. 211–12.

32 Ibid., p. 214.

33 Ibid., p. 216. This study of the results of major operations has relevance to the results of surgical practice given in chapter 8.

34 Ibid., pp. 216–17. Clark's comments about the hospitals in the metropolis confirm Howard's reports about the London hospitals.

35 Ibid., p. 217. Clark discounts any difference in surgical skills in explaining any of the variations in performance.

36 Quoted from a pamphlet by John Bell in J. Gregory, *Additional Memorial to the Managers of the Royal Infirmary*, pp. 324–5.

37 Clark, op. cit., 'Copy of a Letter to Dr. Gregory, from Mr. Russell, Senior Surgeon to the Royal Infirmary Edinburgh, enclosed in a Letter to Dr. Clark', p. 97.

38 Clark, op. cit., pp. 326–7.

39 Ibid., p. 331.

40 Sympson, op. cit., p. 6.

41 Ibid., p. 7.

42 Salisbury General Infirmary, *Auditors Report*, 30 August 1803–31 August 1804.

43 Edinburgh Royal Infirmary, *Minutes*, 30 July 1821.

44 Ibid., 28 January 1822.

45 Edinburgh Royal Infirmary, *Minutes*, 23 September 1822. I am indebted to Mrs P. M. Eaves-Walton, archivist of the Edinburgh Royal Infirmary, for drawing my attention to this information.

46 General Infirmary at Leeds, *Annual Report*, 29 September 1821–29 September 1822.

47 Glasgow Royal Infirmary, *Minutes*, Report of Medical Committee, May 1823.

48 Ibid., Table C.

49 *A Statement of Facts Relative to the Ventilation of the Sheffield Infirmary*, Sheffield 1833, pp. 1–2.

50 Salisbury General Infirmary, *Auditors Report*, 31 August 1831–31 August 1832.

51 The measures undertaken were:
    1. House to be thoroughly fumigated, floors washed every day with a strong solution of chloride of lime.
    2. No more patients to be received until the medical staff reports that the hospital is in a fit state to receive them.
    3. That those who die shall immediately be wrapped in a

coarse cloth with tar and put in a coffin lined with melted pitch and removed upon a bier.

4. That all linen blankets, etc, that have been used about the sick of a disease suspected to be contagious shall be put into a hamper and lowered into the stream of the river before they are washed, and left in the river six hours.

5. That no beds be used but such as are filled with dry meadow hay and that no second patient be laid on a bed on which a former patient has laid.

6. That all blankets and coverlets be sent in succession to the fulling mill and that from this day no beds or bedding that has been used in the Infirmary be used about a fresh patient.

7. That all sponges and poultice cloths be destroyed.

(Quoted in *Salisbury 200 – The Bi-centenary of Salisbury Infirmary, 1766–1966*, p. 29.)

52 Birmingham General Hospital, *Annual Report*, Midsummer 1834–Midsummer 1835.

53 T. Nunneley, *A Treatise on the Nature, Causes, and Treatment of Erysipelas*, p. 143.

54 The point made about hospital-gangrene is of some note as it is normally suggested that this particular form of sepsis did not appear until the end of the 1840s, rising to a peak in the 1860s. T. Nunneley makes the distinction between erysipelas and hospital-gangrene, so they are not being used for the same form of sepsis. Note, the earlier use of the term 'hospital-gangrene' by Dr Gregory at the Edinburgh Royal Infirmary at the beginning of the nineteenth century. See p. 105.

55 N. Chevers, 'An inquiry into certain of the causes of death after injuries and surgical operations in London hospitals', *Guy's Hospital Reports*, 1, 2nd series, 1843, p. 89.

56 Ibid., p. 89.

57 Ibid., p. 102.

58 Ibid., p. 102.

59 T. Bryant, 'On the causes of death after amputation', *Medico-Chirurgical Transactions*, 24, 2nd series, 1859, p. 87.

60 Ibid., p. 87.

61 Birmingham General Hospital, Special Medical Board, 16 March 1859, quoted in *Annual Report*, Midsummer 1858–Midsummer 1859.

62 Birmingham General Hospital, *Annual Report*, Midsummer 1862–Midsummer 1863.

63 'A statement of the views of the weekly board of the general hospital respecting its past and future management', part 1, section 2, quoted in *Annual Report*, Midsummer 1863–Midsummer 1864.

64 Birmingham General Hospital, *Annual Report*, Midsummer 1867–Midsummer 1868.

65 Birmingham General Hospital, *Annual Report*, 1 January 1875–31 December 1875.

66 York County Hospital, *Court of Governors*, 8 September 1846.
67 Ibid., 11 February 1840.
68 *Report of a Committee on the Warming and Ventilation of the York County Hospital*, May 1852, p. 6.
69 York County Hospital, *Proceedings of the House Committee*, 23 March 1858.
70 Ibid., 9 June 1859.
71 Ibid., 11 October 1859.
72 J. S. Bristowe and T. Holmes, *The Hospitals of the United Kingdom*, p. 547. Despite this optimistic statement, there was a recurrence of 'hospital disease' in 1870.
73 *British and Foreign Medico-Chirurgical Review*, 37, 1866, pp. 1–28; and 38, 1866, pp. 370–97.
   (a) A. Husson, *Hospitals Considered with Reference to their Construction, etc.*, Paris, 1862.
   (b) M. M. Blondel & Ser, *Report on the Civil Hospitals of London as Compared with those of Paris*, Paris, 1862.
   (c) A. Uytterhoven, *Notice of the Hospital of St. John. On the best Mode of Constructing and Organising an Hospital for the Sick*, 2nd ed., Brussels, 1862.
   (d) *Discussion on the Hygiene and Salubrity of Hospitals at the Surgical Society of Paris*, Paris, 1865.
   (e) J. Ranald Martin, 'On hospitals' in T. Holmes (ed.), *A System of Surgery*, London, 1864.
   (f) E. Parkes, *A Manual of Practical Hygiene*, London, 1864.
   (g) J. S. Bristowe and T. Holmes, *Hospitals of the United Kingdom*, London, 1864.
   (h) *The Builder*, various articles, London, 1858.
   (i) J. Pozzi, *On Hospitals*, Livorno, 1839.
   (j) F. Nightingale, *Notes on Hospitals*, 3rd ed., London, 1863.
   It should be noted that it was not only the British hospitals which apparently needed attention.
74 J. Simon, *Sixth Report of the Medical Officer of the Privy Council*, 1863, pp. 39–40.
75 F. Nightingale, *Notes on Hospitals*, 3rd ed., 1863.
76 Bristowe and Holmes, op. cit. In addition, the report was commissioned after the controversy over the removal of St Thomas's Hospital to a rural site.
77 Nightingale, op. cit., pp. 26–7.
78 For example, the article by Sir J. Ranald Martin 'On hospitals' in T. Holmes (ed.), *A System of Surgery*, London, 1864.
79 Nightingale, op. cit., p. 56.
80 Bristowe and Holmes, op. cit., p. 478.
81 Ibid., p. 481.
82 Ibid., p. 494.
83 Ibid., p. 491.
84 Ibid., p. 552.
85 Ibid., p. 553.
86 Ibid., p. 554.

o

87 Ibid., p. 554.
88 J. Y. Simpson, 'Hospitalism and its effects, part II', p. 50; reprinted from the *Edinburgh Medical Journal*, 24 June 1869.
89 Ibid., part I, pp. 3–4; reprinted from *Edinburgh Medical Journal*, March 1869.
90 'The accuracy of Sir James Simpson's statistics of the results of amputations in country and private practice has been seriously impugned by Callender, Holmes, and other authorities, owing to the impossibility of proving the reliability of the sources from which they were derived, and because no details of the cases were given' (H. C. Burdett, 'The relative mortality after amputations, of large and small hospitals, and the influence of the antiseptic (Listerian) system upon such mortality', *Journal of the Statistical Society*, 45, September 1882, p. 445).
91 T. Nunneley, 'Address in surgery', *British Medical Journal*, 2, 1869, p. 156 (footnote). A new infirmary had been constructed because of the overcrowding in the old building and the first patient was moved into the new Infirmary on 22 May 1869. (General Infirmary at Leeds, *Annual Report*, 31 December 1868–31 December 1869.)
92 Nunneley, op. cit., p. 156. It is interesting to note that though his colleagues used antiseptic methods Nunneley did not. The use of Listerian techniques will be considered in the final section of this chapter.
93 For example, the discussion on pyaemia in *Clinical Society Transactions*, 7, 1868.
94 *Mr. Netten Radcliffe's Report to the Local Government Board on the Sanitary Condition of the Royal Infirmary*, p. 30. J. Netten Radcliffe was the Secretary of the Epidemiological Society, and had been appointed to one of the two newly-created health inspectorships under Sir John Simon at the Medical Department of the Privy Council in 1869.
95 Ibid., p. 30. Note, in each year during this period the Manchester Royal Infirmary was treating between 2,000 and 3,000 in-patients. Thus, the number of cases of sepsis recorded was a small percentage of the total number admitted to the infirmary.
96 Sympson, op. cit., pp. 13–14.
97 Quoted in ibid., p. 25.
98 J. E. Erichsen, *Hospitalism and the Causes of Death after Operations and Surgical Injuries*, p. 28. Note, the evidence would suggest, however, that the incidence of 'hospital diseases' was liable to fluctuation from one year, or even month, to the next.
99 Ibid., p. 58.
100 For example, Burdett, op. cit., writing in 1882.
101 J. Lister, 'On a new method of treating compound fracture, abscess, etc., with observations on the conditions of suppuration', *Lancet*, 1, 1867.
102 Ibid., p. 327.
103 Ibid., p. 327.

104 J. Lister, 'On the effects of the antiseptic system of treatment upon the salubrity of a surgical hospital', *Lancet*, 1, 1870.
105 T. Holmes and W. B. Holdernesse, 'On the treatment of wounds by the application of carbolic acid, on Lister's method', *St. George's Hospital Reports*, 3, 1868, p. 248.
106 J. Lister, 'Further evidence regarding the effects of the antiseptic system of treatment upon the salubrity of a surgical hospital', *Lancet*, 2, 1870, p. 288.
107 Ibid., p. 288.
108 T. Holmes, 'On the amputation-book of St. George's Hospital, no. II', *St. George's Hospital Reports*, 8, 1874–6, p. 273.
109 Ibid.
110 Ibid., p. 275.

Chapter 10 Gateways to death?

1 T. McKeown and R. G. Brown, 'Medical evidence related to English population changes in the eighteenth century', *Population Studies*, 9, 1955–6, p. 125.
2 Ibid., p. 125.
3 J. Howard, *Account of the Principal Lazarettos in Europe.*
4 J. R. Tenon, *Mémoires sur les Hôpitaux de Paris*, Paris, 1788.
5 W. Woollcombe, *Remarks on the Frequency and Fatality of Different Diseases*, Table VII, Average of deaths at several institutions, pp. 105–6. In the least mortal hospitals (the Devon and Exeter Hospital and the Woolwich Infirmary) the death-rates were as low as one in thirty-five and even in the London hospitals the rate averaged only one in thirteen.
6 J. E. Erichsen, *Hospitalism and the Causes of Death after Operations and Surgical Injuries.*
7 McKeown and Brown, op. cit., p. 120.
8 F. Nightingale, *Notes on Hospitals.*
9 *Medical Times and Gazette*, 30 January 1864, p. 129.
10 Ibid.
11 Ibid.
12 *Medical Times and Gazette*, 13 February 1864, p. 186.
13 *Medical Times and Gazette*, 30 April 1864, p. 491. This criticism was in answer to the calculation made by William Farr that 'while the annual mortality of the general population was 2·16 per cent, the mortality of their [i.e. the hospitals'] inmates was at the rate of 56·87 per cent, or 26 times as high'. Though Dr Farr did have the graciousness to admit that 'The inmates of hospitals, it is scarcely necessary to say, all suffer from diseases which tend generally to increase the risk of death' (W. Farr, 'Letter to the Registrar General on the causes of death in England', appendix to the *24th Annual Report of the Registrar-General of Births, Deaths and Marriages in England*, 1863, p. 230).
14 *Medical Times and Gazette*, 30 April 1864, p. 492.

15   J. S. Bristowe and T. Holmes, *The Hospitals of the United Kingdom*, p. 513.
16   The principal sources of data are the annual reports of the voluntary hospitals, supplemented by various studies and surveys made by interested persons and authorities.
17   Sir W. Petty, *Two Essays in Political Arithmetic concerning the People, Housing, Hospitals &c. of London and Paris*, London, 1687, reprinted in C. H. Hull (ed.), *The Economic Writings of Sir William Petty*, vol. 2, p. 511. These figures were compared favourably with the experience of 'La Charité' in Paris where more than an eighth of the patients admitted died 'which shews that out of the most poor and wretched Hospitals of London there died fewer in proportion than out of the best in Paris' (ibid.).
18   *Spittal Sermon*, Easter Monday, 1726.
19   *Spittal Sermon*, Easter Monday, 1735.
20   'With reference to the class designated "cured" or "well", it is well known to those accustomed to hospital practice, that the meaning intended to be conveyed is not an absolute and permanent recovery from disease in all cases, but that it includes a very large number of cases where a restoration to temporary health is the utmost that can be expected. In fevers and in the greater number of surgical diseases, especially external injuries and patients subjected to operative interference, no doubt can exist as to the credibility of the return "well", the amount of relief afforded must be accepted within circumscribed limits.
     'The same remark is equally applicable to the division "relieved". . . . Under this latter heading are included a large, perhaps the greater portion of the patients whose classification might, with equal propriety, have been inserted in the category of incurable cases, were it not for the fact that they had received benefit from their temporary residence, and were discharged much better in health than they were at the date of their admission' (J. C. Steele, 'Numerical analysis of the patients treated in Guy's Hospital for the last seven years, from 1854 to 1861', *Journal of the Statistical Society*, 24, September 1861, p. 376).
     The classifications given for the middle of the nineteenth century should be compared with the definition of 'relieved' given by the Edinburgh Royal Infirmary in the first half of the eighteenth century – 'Recovery so as to go about their ordinary Affairs and required only some Time to confirm their Health, and to restore their Strength fully' ('An Account of the Rise and Establishment of the Infirmary, or Hospital for Sick-Poor, Erected at Edinburgh, 1730', quoted in J. D. Comrie, *History of Scottish Medicine to 1860*, vol. 2, p. 451).
21   Salisbury General Infirmary, *Annual Report*, 1875–6, 'A General Abstract of the State of the Patients from the First Establishment'.
22   Salisbury General Infirmary, *Annual Report*, 1770–1.
23   Salisbury General Infirmary, *Annual Report*, 1835–6.
24   H. Bevan, *Records of the Salop Infirmary*, no. 2, 'Abstract of In

and Out Patients discharged from the first opening of the Institution, in 1747 to 1846 (inclusive)'.

25 Ibid., no. 3.
26 Manchester Infirmary, *Annual Report*, 1769–70.
27 Manchester Royal Infirmary, *Annual Report*, 1874–5. The overall number of patients treated includes all the types treated, namely, in-patients, out-patients, home-patients, fever and convalescent patients.
28 Bristol Infirmary, *Annual Reports*, 1811 and 1828.
29 Liverpool Infirmary, *Annual Report*, 1760–1.
30 Liverpool Infirmary, *Annual Report*, 1875.
31 Annual reports of the Royal Infirmaries at Edinburgh and Glasgow to 1875.
32 St Thomas's Hospital, *Annual Reports*, 1786–90 and 1870–6.
33 G. Blane, 'On the comparative prevalence and mortality of different diseases in London', *Medico-Chirurgical Transactions*, 1, 1813, p. 142.
34 J. Clark, *A Collection of Papers, intended to promote An Institution for the Cure and Prevention of Infectious Fevers*, supplement, p. 216. These figures were produced as part of a campaign to build a fever house and to improve sanitary conditions at the Newcastle Infirmary. The figures used were subsequently reproduced in a survey of disease published in 1808: W. Woollcombe, *The Frequency and Fatality of Different Diseases*.
35 D. Phelan, *A Statistical Enquiry into the Present State of the Medical Charities of Ireland*, Table no. VII, A statistical report of the principal provincial hospitals in England (abbreviated from the Rev. Mr. Oxenden's report) – hospital-year, 1830.
36 G. R. Porter, *The Progress of the Nation*, section 1, p. 41.
37 Ibid., p. 42.
38 *A Comparative Statement of the Economy of Thirty-Two Provincial Hospitals and Infirmaries*, compiled by a member of the Committee of Birmingham General, 1844.
39 F. Buckle, *Vital and Economical Statistics of the Hospitals, Infirmaries Etc. of England and Wales for the Year 1863*.
40 Ibid., Table no. 1: 'no "bed-rate" has been given, as it is obvious that in many country hospitals, where perhaps only half the number of beds are occupied at a time, the rate would be much lower than it should be, while in others, where the beds are constantly full, it would be correspondingly high.'
41 Bristowe and Holmes, op. cit., p. 569.
42 Ibid., p. 513.
43 Ibid., p. 513.
44 London Hospital, *Annual Report*, 1 January 1795–1 January 1796.
45 London Hospital, *Annual Report*, 1 January 1833–1 January 1834.
46 Bristowe and Holmes, op. cit., p. 513 (footnote).
47 Ibid.
48 Sheffield Royal Infirmary, *Annual Report*, Midsummer 1844– Midsummer 1845.

49   Sheffield Royal Infirmary, *Minute of the Weekly Board*, 9 February 1848; quoted in *Annual Report*, Midsummer 1847–Midsummer 1848.
50   Sheffield Royal Infirmary, *Annual Report*, Midsummer 1854–Midsummer 1855.
51   Salisbury General Infirmary, *Annual Report*, 31 August 1845–29 August 1846.
52   Bristowe and Holmes, op. cit., p. 514.
53   General Infirmary at Leeds, *Annual Report*, 1786.
54   Bristowe and Holmes, op. cit., p. 514, footnote.
55   Ibid., pp. 516–17.
56   Ibid., p. 516, Table.
57   Ibid.
58   Ibid., p. 517.
59   Ibid., footnote. It was not possible to measure the proportion of beds allocated to medical and surgical cases generally before the middle years of the nineteenth century as it took until this late date for all hospitals to recognize the desirability of separating their patients, although this had been advocated in the eighteenth century by such reformers as John Howard.
60   Ibid., p. 518.
61   J. C. Steele, 'The mortality of hospitals, general and special, in the United Kingdom, in times past and present', *Journal of the Statistical Society*, 40, 1877, p. 196.
62   Ibid., pp. 196–7.
63   Ibid., p. 197.
64   Bristowe and Holmes, op. cit., p. 520.
65   Ibid.
66   Steele, 'The mortality of hospitals . . .', p. 207.
67   Ibid., pp. 212–13.
68   Bristowe and Holmes, op. cit., p. 521.
69   Ibid., p. 522.
70   Glasgow Royal Infirmary, *Annual Report*, 1846.
71   Manchester Royal Infirmary, *Annual Report*, 25 June 1860–24 June 1861.
72   Bristowe and Holmes, op. cit., p. 523.
73   Liverpool Infirmary, *Annual Report*, 1802. A separate building for the treatment of venereal patients had been established by Liverpool Infirmary in 1772.
74   Devon and Exeter Hospital, *Annual Reports*.
75   Bristowe and Holmes, op. cit., pp. 524–5. In the large hospitals of London and the provinces specific mention was made in the annual reports of the 'trivial cases' which were treated as out-patients, but which were excluded from the computation. For example, the Liverpool Infirmary stated that it had not included in its calculations 'a great number who have been relieved by Bleeding, drawing Teeth, &c., as well as Medicine dispensed for many poor Children inoculated for the Small-pox' (*Annual Report*, 7 March 1785–6 March 1786). Note, chapter 5 deals with the question of the admittance of chronic cases.

76   See the section on medical education (pp. 23–6).
77   Bristowe and Holmes, op. cit., p. 526.
78   See chapter 9.
79   Bristowe and Holmes, op. cit., p. 567.
80   Bevan, op. cit., Table no. 6 – 'A comparative statement, showing the average number of days which each patient of the Salop Infirmary, remained in the house at different periods'.
81   Phelan, op. cit., Rev. Oxenden's report.
82   Buckle, op. cit., Table 1.
83   R. Pinker, *English Hospital Statistics 1861–1938*.
84   It is assumed by Pinker that the details given by Buckle for 1863 and Bristowe and Holmes for 1862 were not significantly different from those for 1861.
85   Pinker, op. cit., Table xxiv, p. 114.
86   Ibid., Table xxv, p. 119.
87   Ibid., p. 118. The low figure recorded for the hospital at Bath is a repetition of earlier experience at this institution.
88   Ibid., pp. 120–2.
89   Hull Royal Infirmary, *Annual Reports*, 1864 to 1874.
90   Glasgow Royal Infirmary, *Annual Report*, 1875.
91   Bristowe and Holmes, op. cit., p. 536.
92   Ibid.
93   Ibid., p. 527. Robert Lawson Tait in his essay on hospital mortality in 1877 made a similar comment on the possible adjustment of the figures so it would appear that the practice was not unknown even at this late date (R. Lawson Tait, *An Essay on Hospital Mortality*, p. 11).
94   *Oxford Journal*, 9 December 1786.
95   Quoted in H. J. C. Gibson, *Dundee Royal Infirmary 1798 to 1948*, pp. 19–20. Mr Munro, the surgeon, had performed forty-nine operations in the previous year without any fatal results, twenty-four amputations had been performed and some of the cases were 'of considerable gravity'. He also made the comment that his success had 'not arisen in the slightest degree from any exclusion of patients in consequence of their being incurable or otherwise unfit objects of admission' (ibid.).
96   Bristowe and Holmes, op. cit., p. 527.
97   Lawson Tait, op. cit., p. 10. In this chapter the figures given have been based on the numbers completing their treatment within the hospital-year. Patients in the hospital at the beginning and end of the year were given in the annual reports and allowance has been made for these cases.
98   Bristowe and Holmes, op. cit., p. 527.
99   Lawson Tait, op. cit., pp. 10–11.
100 Leicester Infirmary, *Annual Report*, 1870.
101 Leicester Infirmary, *Annual Report*, 1875.
102 Bristowe and Holmes, op. cit., p. 527.
103 Lawson Tait, op. cit., p. 11.

Chapter 11 Hospitals and population growth

1 T. McKeown and R. G. Brown, 'Medical evidence related to English population changes in the eighteenth century', *Population Studies*, 9, 1955–6, p. 125.

2 P. Deane, *The First Industrial Revolution*, 1965, p. 29.

3 P. Mathias, *The First Industrial Nation*, 1969, p. 189.

4 K. F. Helleiner, 'The vital revolution reconsidered', *Canadian Journal of Economic and Political Science*, no. 1, 1957; reprinted in D. V. Glass and D. E. C. Eversley (eds), *Population in History*, p. 84.

5 Additional changes in medical treatment for the poor during the eighteenth century, namely, the development of dispensaries and the practice of inoculation against smallpox, will be discussed later in this chapter.

6 'The London Bills of Mortality have long been deemed incorrect, and indeed very justly; the reports being generally taken from the nurses, or ignorant domestics, who are frequently unacquainted with the proper names and distinctions of the diseases recorded in those yearly accounts' (J. C. Lettsom, *Medical Memoirs of the General Dispensary in London for Part of the Years 1773 and 1774*, pp. 343–4).

7 T. Short, *New Observations Natural, Moral, Civil, Political and Medical, on City, Town and Country Bills of Mortality. To which are added Large and Clear Abstracts of the best Authors, who have wrote on that subject. With an Appendix on the Weather and Meteors*, p. 176; quoted in T. H. Hollingsworth, *Historical Demography*, p. 146. It was stated that half of the burial places which had not been taken account of belonged to the Established Church.

8 J. K. Edwards, 'Norwich Bills of Mortality – 1707–1830', *Yorkshire Bulletin of Economic and Social Research*, 21, 1969, p. 103.

9 O. Allen, *History of the York Dispensary*, p. 2.

10 W. Hartston, 'Medical dispensaries in eighteenth century London', *Proceedings of the Royal Society of Medicine — Section of the History of Medicine*, 56, 1963, p. 757.

11 Lettsom, op. cit., p. 11.

12 P. E. Razzell, 'Population change in eighteenth century England: a re-appraisal', *Economic History Review*, 18, 1965, p. 331.

13 An examination of the work of the Norfolk and Norwich Hospital concluded: 'Thus, the hospital may have made a partial contribution to falling mortality rates in Norwich in the late eighteenth century, although improved living standards were essential before mortality rates could be reduced permanently. In the early nineteenth century the work of the hospital was countered by economic recession and inadequate public health measures, which, in the face of heavy population growth, worsened poverty and the incidence of disease. At best the hospital may now only have been able to help hold mortality rates at existing levels, rather than to reduce them

further. It may be significant that in the period 1840–80 mortality rates in the city did not fall appreciably' (S. Cherry, 'The role of a provincial hospital: the Norfolk and Norwich Hospital, 1771–1880', *Population Studies*, 26, 1972, p. 305).

Bibliography

Books and pamphlets

Abel-Smith, B., *A History of the Nursing Profession*, Heinemann, London, 1960.

Abel-Smith, B., *The Hospitals 1800–1948*, Heinemann, London, 1964.

Aikin, J., *Thoughts on Hospitals*, J. Johnson, London, 1771.

Allen, O., *History of the York Dispensary*, York, 1845.

Anning, S. T., *The General Infirmary at Leeds . . .* , vols 1 and 2, E. & S. Livingstone, Edinburgh and London, 1963.

Anon., *A Short Answer to a Late Book*, London, 1705.

Barrow, J., *A New Medicinal Dictionary*, T. Longman & C. Hitch; A. Miller, London, 1749.

Bateman, T., *A Practical Synopsis of Cutaneous Diseases*, 3rd ed., Longman & Co., London, 1814.

Bayly, E., *A Short Account of the Nature, Rise and Progress of the General Infirmary at Bath*, Leake, Bath, 1749.

Bellers, J., *An Essay Towards The Improvement of Physick in Twelve Proposals*, The Assigns of J. Sowle, London, 1714.

Bevan, H., *Records of the Salop Infirmary from the commencement of the charity to the present time, being a period of one hundred years*, Sandford & Howell, Shrewsbury, 1847.

Bickerton, T. H., *A Medical History of Liverpool from the Earliest Days to the Year 1920*, John Murray, London, 1936.

Bishop, W. J., *The Early History of Surgery*, R. Hale, London, 1960.

Black, W., *Observations Medical and Political on the Small-Pox and Inoculation*, J. Johnson, London, 1781.

Blizard, W., *Suggestions for the Improvement of Hospitals and Other Charitable Institutions*, C. Dilly, London, 1796.

Bloomfield, J., *St. George's 1733–1933*, Medici Society, London, 1933.

Bosanquet, S. R., *The Rights of the Poor and Christian Almsgiving Vindicated*, James Burns, London, 1841.

Brockbank, W., *Portrait of a Hospital 1752–1948*, Heinemann, London, 1952.

Brockbank, W., *The History of Nursing at the Manchester Royal Infirmary*, Manchester University Press, 1970.

Brockington, C. F., *A Short History of Public Health*, J. & A. Churchill, London, 1966.

Brocklesby, T., *Oeconomical and Medical Observations*, T. Becket & P. A. De Hondt, London, 1764.

Buchanan, M. S., *History of Glasgow Royal Infirmary*, Lumsden, Glasgow, 1832.

202

Buckle, F., *Vital and Economical Statistics of the Hospitals, Infirmaries Etc. of England and Wales for the Year 1863*, J. Churchill, London, 1865.

Buer, M. C., *Health, Wealth, and Population*, G. Routledge, London, 1926.

Bunce, J. T., *A History of the Birmingham General Hospital and the Music Festivals*, Cornish Bros, Birmingham, 1873.

Cannings, R. B., *The City of London Maternity Hospital*, London, 1922.

Cartwright, F. F., *The Development of Modern Surgery*, A. Barker, London, 1967.

Chalmers, A. K., *The Health of Glasgow 1818–1925 – An Outline*, Glasgow Corporation, 1930.

Champney, T., *A Review of the Healing Art*, J. Johnson, London, 1797.

Chaplin, A., *Medicine in the Reign of George III*, London, 1919.

Chelius, J. M., *A System of Surgery* (trans. J. F. South), Henry Renshaw, London, 1847.

Cheselden, W., *The Anatomy of the Humane Body*, 7th ed., C. Hitch & R. Dodsley, London, 1756.

Christisons, *The Life of Sir Robert Christison, Bart*, W. Slackwood & Sons, Edinburgh, 1885.

Clare, P., *An Essay on the Cure of Abscesses by Caustic*, T. Cadell, London, 1779.

Clark, J., *A Collection of Papers, intended to promote An Institution for the Cure and Prevention of Infectious Fevers in Newcastle and other Populous Towns*, S. Hodgson, Newcastle, 1802.

Clark-Kennedy, A. E., *The London – A Study in the Voluntary Hospital System*, vols 1 and 2, Pitman, London, 1962.

Clarke, A., *Sermon, October 18, 1736. To which is added a collection of papers, rules, and orders relating to the rise, progress, and government of this charity*, (*Winchester County Hospital*), 3rd ed., William Chase, Norwich, 1769.

Clarke, E. (ed.), *Modern Methods in the History of Medicine*, Athlone Press, London, 1973.

Clay, R. M., *The Medieval Hospitals of England*, Methuen, London, 1909.

Clendenning, L., *Source Book of Medical History*, Hoeber, New York, 1942.

Coates, W. M., *On Chloroform and Its Safe Administration*, Walton & Maberly, London and Salisbury, 1858.

Comrie, J. D., *History of Scottish Medicine to 1860*, vols 1 and 2, Wellcome, London, 1927.

Cook, E. T., *Life of Florence Nightingale*, Macmillan, London, 1925.

Copeman, E., *Brief History of the Norfolk and Norwich Hospital*, Norwich, 1856.

Cowan, R., *Statistics of Fever and Small-Pox in Glasgow*, David Robertson, Glasgow, 1837.

Crosse, V. M., *A Surgeon in the Early Nineteenth Century*, E. & S. Livingstone, Edinburgh and London, 1968.

Davidson, M., *Medicine in Oxford*, Blackwell, Oxford, 1953.

De Laune, T., *Angliae Metropolis: or the present state of London*, George Larkin for John Harris & Thomas Howkins, London, 1690.

Duncum, B. M., *The Development of Inhalation Anaesthesia. With special reference to the years 1846–1900*, Wellcome, London, 1947.

Duncumb, J., *A Sermon preached in the cathedral church of Hereford on Thursday, the third of August 1797, at the annual meeting of the subscribers to the General Infirmary in that city*, D. Walker, Hereford, 1797.

Eade, Sir P., *The Norfolk and Norwich Hospital 1779–1900*, Jarrold, London, 1900.

Eaves-Walton, P. M., *Royal Infirmary of Edinburgh 1729–1900*, E.R.I., Edinburgh, 1968.

Enfield, W., *An Essay Towards the History of Liverpool*, J. Johnson, London, 1774.

Erichsen, J. E., *Hospitalism and the Causes of Death after Operations and Surgical Injuries*, Longmans, Green, London, 1874.

Ernest, R., *A Synopsis of Medical and Surgical Cases at the Sheffield General Infirmary During Twenty-Two Years*, C. &. W. Thompson, Sheffield, 1820.

Farmer, L., *Master Surgeon – A Biography of Joseph Lister*, Harper, New York, 1962.

Ferriar, J., *Medical Histories and Reflections*, Cadell & Davies, London, Warrington, 1810–13.

Fleetwood, J., *History of Medicine in Ireland*, Browne & Nolan, Dublin, 1951.

Forbes, J., *et al.* (eds), *The Cyclopaedia of Practical Medicine*, Sherwood, Gilbert & Piper, London, 1835.

Foster, W. D., *A Short History of Clinical Pathology*, Livingstone, Edinburgh and London, 1961.

Foy, G., *Anaesthetics, Ancient and Modern*, Baillière, London, 1889.

Frith, B., *The Story of Gloucester's Infirmary*, Gloucester H.M.C., Gloucester, 1961.

Frizelle, E. R. and Martin, J. D., *The Leicester Royal Infirmary 1771–1971*, Leicester No. 1 H.M.C., Leicester, 1971.

Garth, S., *Oratoria Laudatoria*, London, 1697.

Gaskell, P., *Artisans and Machinery*, John W. Parker, London, 1836.

George, M. D., *London Life in the Eighteenth Century*, 3rd ed., L.S.E., London, 1951.

George, M. D., *England in Transition*, Penguin, London, 1962.

Gibson, A. G., *The Radcliffe Infirmary*, Oxford University Press, Oxford and London, 1926.

Gibson, H. J. C., *Dundee Royal Infirmary 1798 to 1948*, W. Kidd, Dundee, 1948.

Gibson, J., *Great Doctors and Medical Scientists*, Macmillan, London, 1967.

Glass, D. V. and Eversley, D. E. C. (eds), *Population in History*, Arnold, London, 1965.

Golding, B., *An Historical Account of St. Thomas's Hospital, Southwark*, Longman, London, 1819.

Graham, H., *Surgeons All*, 2nd ed., Rich & Cowan, London, 1956.

Greenwood, M., *Some British Pioneers of Social Medicine*, Oxford University Press, London, 1948.

Grey, R., *The Encouragement to Works of Charity and Mercy . . .*, W. Dicey, Northampton, 1744.

Guthrie, D., *A History of Medicine*, T. Nelson, London, 1960.

Hall, J. M. and Harral, V. C., *The General Hospital, Birmingham*, U.B.H., Birmingham, 1967.

Halton, J. P., *The Results of the Great Operations of Surgery . . .*, Liverpool, 1843.

Harris, J. D., *The Royal Devon and Exeter Hospital*, Eland, Exeter, 1922.

Hartlib, S., *A Description of the Famous Kingdome of Macaria*, London, 1641.

Haskins, C., *The History of Salisbury Infirmary*, Salisbury Times, Salisbury, 1922.

Haslam, W. F., *A Review of the Operations for Stone in the Male Bladder*, Harrison & Sons, London, 1911.

Hawkins, C. (ed.), *The Works of Sir Benjamin Brodie*, vols 1 and 2, Longmans, London, 1865.

Hawkins, F. B., *Elements of Medical Statistics*, Longman, London, 1829.

Heberden, W., *Observations on the Increase and Decrease of Different Diseases, and Particularly of the Plague*, London, 1801.

Highmore, A., *Pietas Londiniensis: The History, Design and Present State of the Various Public Charities In and Near London*, Cradock & Joy, London, 1810.

Hill, A. W., *John Wesley Among the Physicians – A Study of 18th Century Medicine*, Epworth Press, London, 1958.

Hodgkinson, R. G., *The Origins of the National Health Service – The Medical Services of the New Poor Law 1834–1871*, Wellcome, London, 1967.

Holland, G. C., *The Vital Statistics of Sheffield*, R. Tyas, London, 1843.

Hollingsworth, T. H., *Historical Demography*, Cornell University Press, London, 1969.

Holmes, T. (ed.), *A System of Surgery*, vols 1–14, Longmans, Green & Co., London, 1864.

Howard, J., *The State of the Prisons in England and Wales*, 2nd ed., W. Eyres, Warrington, 1780.

Howard, J., *An Account of the Principal Lazarettos in Europe*, W. Eyres for T. Cadell, Warrington, 1789.

Hull, C. H. (ed.), *The Economic Writings of Sir William Petty*, New York, 1964.

Humble, J. G. and Hansell, P., *Westminster Hospital 1716–1966*, Pitman, London, 1966.

Hume, G. H., *The History of the Newcastle Infirmary*, Andrew Reid & Co., Newcastle-upon-Tyne, 1906.

Hume, W. E., *The Infirmary, Newcastle-upon-Tyne 1751–1951 – A brief sketch*, Andrew Reid, Newcastle-upon-Tyne, 1951.

Humphreys, N. A. (ed.), *Vital Statistics – a memorial volume of selections from the reports and writings of W. Farr*, Royal Society for the Promotion of Health, London, 1885.

Ives, A. G. L., *British Hospitals*, Collins, London, 1948.

Jacob, F. H., *A History of the General Hospital near Nottingham*, Wright, Bristol and London, 1951.

James, R., *A Medicinal Dictionary*, vols 1–3, printed for T. Osborne, London, 1743–5.

Kirkland, T., *Observations upon Mr. Pott's General Remarks on Fractures &c.*, T. Becket & P. A. De Hondt, London, 1770.

Lancet, *The Lancet Commission on Nursing – The Final Report*, London, 1932.

Langdon-Brown, W., *Some Chapters in Cambridge Medical History*, Cambridge University Press, 1946.

Langdon-Davies, J., *Westminster Hospital, 1719–1948*, Murray, London, 1952.

Leader, J. D. and Snell, S., *Sheffield Royal Infirmary, 1797–1897*, Sheffield Infirmary, 1897.

Lettsom, J. C., *Medical Memoirs of the General Dispensary in London for Part of the Years 1773 and 1774*, E. & C. Dilley, London, 1774.

Lister, J., *The Collected Papers of Joseph Baron Lister*, vols 1 and 2, Clarendon Press, Oxford, 1909.

Low, S., *The Charities of London in 1861*, S. Low, London, 1862.

Lowson, K. J. and Grieve, R., *The Story of the Hull Royal Infirmary 1782–1948*, H.R.I., Hull, 1948.

McDougal, J. W., *The Dumfries and Galloway Royal Infirmary – A Brief Pictorial Survey, 1776–1948*, Grieve, Dumfries, 1948.

McInnes, E. M., *St Thomas's Hospital*, Allen & Unwin, London, 1963.

Mackenzie, T. C., *The Royal Northern Infirmary – Inverness – The Story of a Scottish Voluntary Hospital*, R.N.I., Inverness, 1946.

McKeown, T., *Medicine in Modern Society*, Allen & Unwin, London, 1965.

McLachlan, G. and McKeown, T. (eds), *Medical History and Medical Care*, Oxford University Press, London, 1971.

McMenemey, W. H., *A History of the Worcester Royal Infirmary*, Press Alliances, Worcester and London, 1947.

Maddox, I., *The Duty and Advantages of Encouraging Public Infirmaries*, 3rd ed., J. Brotherton, London, 1743.

Marcet, A., *An Essay on the Chemical History and Medical Treatment of Calculous Disorders*, Longman, London, 1817.

Mathias, P., *Science and Society, 1600–1900*, Cambridge University Press, London, 1972.

Medical Society of Observation, *Statistical Reports of Amputations, Compound Fractures, Operations for Hernia and Lithotomy in London Hospitals*, London, 1841.

Miller, A., *An Inquiry into the Average Mortality in Lithotomy Cases: with a few remarks on the operation of lithotrity*, A. Shortreed, Edinburgh, 1831.

Mitchell, B. R. and Deane, P., *Abstract of British Historical Statistics*, Cambridge University Press, 1962.

Moore, Sir N., *The History of St Bartholomew's Hospital*, vols 1 and 2, Pearson, London, 1918.

Mouat, F. J. and Snell, H. S., *Hospital Construction and Management*, J. & A. Churchill, London, 1883.

Munro-Smith, G., *A History of the Bristol Royal Infirmary*, Arrowsmith, Bristol and London, 1917.

Murchison, C., *A Treatise on the Continued Fevers of Great Britain*, 2nd ed., Longmans, Green, London, 1873.

Newman, C., *The Evolution of Medical Education in the Nineteenth Century*, Oxford University Press, London, 1957.

Newman, G., *Health and Social Evolution*, Allen & Unwin, London, 1931.

Nightingale, F., *Notes on Hospitals*, 3rd ed., London, 1863.

Nunneley, T., *A Treatise on the Nature, Causes, and Treatment of Erysipelas*, J. Churchill, London and Leeds, 1841.

Nunneley, T., *Operations Performed at the General Infirmary at Leeds*, Leeds, 1870.

Owen, D., *English Philanthropy 1660–1960*, Belknap Press, Cambridge (Mass.) and London, 1965.

Parker, G., *The Early History of Surgery in Great Britain*, A. & C. Black, London, 1920.

Parkes, E. A., *A Manual of Practical Hygiene*, John Churchill & Sons, London, 1864.

Patrick, J., *A Short History of Glasgow Royal Infirmary*, Glasgow Infirmary, 1940.

Peachey, G. C., *History of St. George's Hospital*, Bale & Danielson, London, 1910–14.

Percival, T., *Essays Medical, Philosophical, and Experimental*, 4th ed., vols 1 and 2, W. Eyres, Warrington and London, 1789.

Percival, T., *Medical Ethics*, J. Jackson, Manchester, 1803; London, 1827.

Phelan, D., *A Statistical Enquiry into the Present State of the Medical Charities of Ireland*, Hodges & Smith, Dublin, 1835.

Philip, A. P. W., *Some Observations on the Principles which insure the most beneficial exercise of the Medical Profession, both in private practice and public institutions; illustrated by the state of the profession in The City of Worcester during the last twenty years*, W. Walcott, Worcester, 1820.

Pinker, R., *English Hospital Statistics 1861–1938*, Heinemann, London, 1966.

Pitt, R., *The Craft and Frauds of Physick Expos'd*, 2nd ed., T. Childe, London, 1703.

Poland, J., *A Retrospect of Surgery during the Past Century*, Smith, Elder, London, 1901.

Pollak, K. and Underwood, E. A., *The Healers – The Doctor, then and now*, Nelson, London, 1968.

Porter, G. R., *The Progress of the Nation*, C. Knight, London, 1836.

Poynter, F. N. L. (ed.), *The Evolution of Medical Education in Britain*, Pitman, London, 1966.

Poynter, F. N. L. (ed.), *The Evolution of Hospitals in Britain*, Pitman, London, 1968.

Poynter, F. N. L. and Keele, K. D., *A Short History of Medicine*, Mills & Boon, London, 1961.

Pringle, J., *Observations on the Nature and Cure of Hospital and Jayl-Fevers*, A. Millar & D. Wilson, London, 1750.

Pye, C., *A Brief Account of the General Hospital near Birmingham*, Birmingham, 1820.

Renaud, F., *A Short History of the Rise and Progress of the Manchester Royal Infirmary from the Year 1752 to 1877*, Cornish, Manchester, 1898.

Riddell, J. S., *The Records of the Aberdeen Medico-Chirurgical Society from 1789 to 1922*, Lindsay, Aberdeen, 1922.

Ripman, H. A., *Guy's Hospital 1725–1948*, Guy's Hospital Gazette Committee, London, 1951.

Robb-Smith, A. H. T., *A Short History of the Radcliffe Infirmary*, United Oxford Hospitals, Oxford, 1970.

Roux, P. J., *A Narrative of a Journey to London in 1814; or, a parallel of the English and French surgery; preceded by some observations on the London hospitals*, 2nd ed., E. Cox & Son, London, 1816.

Royal College of Physicians of London, *A Picture of the Present State of the Royal College of Physicians of London*, Sherwood, Weeley & Jones, London, 1817.

Rumsey, H. W., *Some Fallacies of Statistics*, Smith, Elder, London, 1875.

Salisbury General Hospital, *Salisbury 200 – The Bi-centenary of Salisbury Infirmary, 1766–1966*, Salisbury General Hospital, Salisbury, 1967.

Saunders, C. J. G., *A History of the United Bristol Hospitals*, United Bristol Hospitals, Bristol, 1965.

Saunders, H. St G., *The Middlesex Hospital 1745–1948*, Parrish, London, 1949.

Seymer, L. R., *A General History of Nursing*, Faber & Faber, London, 1932.

Sheffield City Libraries, *The Sheffield Hospitals*, Local History Leaflets, no. 7, 1959.

Shepherdson, W., *Reminiscences of the Hull General Infirmary*, London and Hull, 1873.

Sinclair, H. M. and Robb-Smith, A. H. T., *A History of the Teaching of Anatomy in Oxford*, Oxford, 1950.

Singer, C. and Underwood, E. A., *A Short History of Medicine*, Oxford University Press, London, 1962.

Snow, J., *On the Inhalation of the Vapour of Ether*, John Churchill, London, 1847; *British Journal of Anaesthesia*, 23, 1953.

Stevens, R., *Medical Practice in Modern England*, Yale University Press, New Haven and London, 1966.

Stonhouse, J., *Friendly Advice To a Patient*, 9th ed., J. Rivington, London, 1750.

Surtz, E. and Hexter, J. H. (eds), *The Complete Works of St Thomas More*, Yale University Press, New Haven and London, 1965.

Sympson, T., *A Short Account of the Old and of the New Lincoln County Hospitals*, J. Williamson, London, 1878.

Tait, R. L., *An Essay on Hospital Mortality*, Churchill, London, 1877.

Thackrah, C. T., *The Effects of Arts, Trades and Professions on Health and Longevity*, Longman, London, 1832; reprinted Edinburgh and London, 1957.

Turner, A. L., *The Royal Infirmary of Edinburgh – Bicentenary Year 1729–1929*, Oliver & Boyd, Edinburgh, 1929.

Turner, A. L., *Story of a Great Hospital: the Royal Infirmary of Edinburgh, 1729–1929*, Oliver & Boyd, Edinburgh, 1937.

University of Edinburgh, *Bicentenary of the Faculty of Medicine 1726–1926*, Edinburgh, 1926.

Walker, J. K., *Observations on the Expediency of Establishing Hospitals*, Huddersfield, 1828.

White, C., *Treatise on the Management of Pregnant and Lying-In Women*, 3rd ed., E. & C. Dilly, London, 1795.

Whitteridge, G. and Stokes, V., *A Brief History of the Hospital of St. Bartholomew*, The Governors of the Hospital of St Bartholomew, London, 1961.

Wilks, S. and Bettany, G. T., *A Biographical History of Guy's Hospital*, Ward, Lock, London, 1892.

Willan, R., *Reports of the Diseases in London Particularly during the Years 1796, '97, '98, '99, and 1800*, R. Phillips, London, 1801.

Willcock, J. W., *The Laws Relating to the Medical Profession*, A. Strahan for J. & W. T. Clarke, London, 1830.

Wilson, E., *The History of the Middlesex Hospital during the first century of its existence compiled from the hospital records*, Churchill, London, 1845.

Withington, E. T., *Medical History from the earliest times*, Scientific Press, London, 1964.

Woodham-Smith, C., *Florence Nightingale*, Constable, London, 1950.

Woollcombe, W., *Remarks on the Frequency and Fatality of Different Diseases*, Longmans, London, 1808.

Yelloly, J., *Remarks on the Tendency to Calculous Diseases*, R. Taylor, London, 1829.

Yelloly, J., *On the Tendency to Calculous Diseases and on the Concretions to which such Diseases give rise*, R. Taylor, London, 1830.

Zimmerman, L. M. and Veith, I. (eds), *Great Ideas in the History of Surgery*, Williams & Witkin, Baltimore, 1961.

Articles

Anning, S. T., 'A hospital pharmacopoeia of the nineteenth century', *Medical History*, 10, 1966.

Anon., 'Statistical analysis of 186 lithotomy operations', *Medical Times and Gazette*, 18 (new series), 1859.

P

Anon., 'Report of the committee on the uses and effects of chloroform', *Medico-Chirurgical Transactions*, 47, 1864.

Anon., 'On the necessity for separate wards for fever cases in general hospitals', *Lancet*, 11 February 1865.

Anon., 'History of Aberdeen Royal Infirmary – its rise and progress', *People's Journal* (Dundee), 1904.

Anon., 'The origin and evolution of the 18th century hospital movement', *Hospital*, nos 10 and 11, 1913–14.

Anon., 'The beginnings of the London Hospital: A new light on its early days', *Hospital*, 11, 1914.

Anon., 'London's earliest health centre', *Chemist and Druggist*, 167, 15, 1951.

Bernard, T., 'Extracts from a further account of the House of Recovery at Manchester', *The Reports of the Society for Bettering the Condition and Increasing the Comforts of the Poor*, 2, 1805.

Blane, Sir G., 'On the comparative prevalence and mortality of different diseases in London', *Medico-Chirurgical Transactions*, 1, 1813.

Bryant, T., 'On the causes of death after amputation', *Medico-Chirurgical Transactions*, 24, 2nd series, 1859.

Bryant, T., 'Contributions to the subject of compound fracture; being an analysis of 302 cases', *Medico-Chirurgical Transactions*, 44, 1861.

Bryant, T., 'An analysis of 230 cases of lithotomy', *Medico-Chirurgical Transactions*, 45, 1862.

Burdett, H. C., 'The relative mortality after amputations, of large and small hospitals', *Journal of the Statistical Society*, September 1882.

Bush, J. P., 'Early history of the Bristol Royal Infirmary', *Bristol Medico-Chirurgical Journal*, September, 1908.

Callender, G. W., 'Some account of the amputations performed at St. Bartholomew's Hospital – from the 1st January 1853 to the 1st October 1863', *Medico-Chirurgical Transactions*, 47, 1864.

Callender, G. W., 'Comparison of the death-rates after amputations in country private practice, in hospital practice, and on country patients in a town hospital', *St. Bartholomew's Hospital Reports*, 5, 1869.

Callender, G. W., 'Note on the death-rate after amputations in hospital practice', *St. Bartholomew's Hospital Reports*, 8, 1872.

Callender, G. W., 'Two years of hospital practice', *St. Bartholomew's Hospital Reports*, 9, 1873.

Carbutt, E., 'Comparative statement of diseases in hospital practice, during four years, viz the years 1826, 1827, 1828, 1829, with observations', *North of England Medical and Surgical Journal*, 1, 1830.

Cherry, S., 'The role of a provincial hospital: the Norfolk and Norwich Hospital, 1771–1880', *Population Studies*, 26, 1972.

Chevers, N., 'An inquiry into certain of the causes of death after injuries and surgical operations in London hospitals', *Guy's Hospital Reports*, 1, 2nd series, 1843.

Cheyne, W. W., 'Statistical report of all operations performed on healthy joints in hospital practice by Mr. Lister from September 1871', *British Medical Journal*, 29 November 1879.

Churchill, E. D., 'The pandemic of wound infection in hospitals', *Journal of the History of Medicine*, 20, 1965.

Civis Academias Edinensis, 'Mortality after lithotomy', *British Medical Journal*, 1, 1879.

Coote, H., 'On lithotomy and lithotrity', *St. Bartholomew's Hospital Reports*, 4, 1868.

Eason, Sir H. (ed.), 'The Steele diaries', *Guy's Hospital Gazette*, 1947, 1948.

Eaves-Walton, P. M., 'The Royal Infirmary of Edinburgh', *Hospital Management*, March, 1968.

Edwards, J. K., 'Norwich Bills of Mortality – 1707–1830', *Yorkshire Bulletin of Economic and Social Research*, 21, November, 1969.

Elcock, C. E., 'Hospital building – past, present and future', *Proceedings of the Royal Society of Medicine – Section of the History of Medicine*, 35, 1941.

Fox, E. L., 'Where should typhus be treated?', *Edinburgh Medical Journal*, January 1866.

Guy, W. A., 'On the mortality of London hospitals', *Journal of the Statistical Society*, 30, 1867.

Hall, I. V., 'The Garlicks, Two generations of a Bristol family (1692–1781)', *Transactions of the Bristol and Gloucestershire Archaeological Society*, 80, 1961.

Hartston, W., 'Medical dispensaries in eighteenth century London', *Proceedings of the Royal Society of Medicine – Section of the History of Medicine*, 56, 1963.

Hartston, W., 'Care of the sick poor in England 1572–1948', *Proceedings of the Royal Society of Medicine – Section of the History of Medicine*, 59, 1966.

Holloway, S. W. F., 'Medical education in England: 1830–1858: a sociological analysis', *History*, 49, 1964.

Holmes, T., 'On the amputation book of St. George's Hospital', *St. George's Hospital Reports*, 1, 1866.

Holmes, T., 'On the influence exerted by treatment in hospitals upon the event of surgical operations and accidents', *British Medical Journal*, 2, 1866.

Holmes, T., 'On the amputation book of St. George's Hospital, no. II. Founded on the notes of five hundred cases there recorded. With some observations on the antiseptic treatment of cases of amputation', *St. George's Hospital Reports*, 8, 1874–6.

Holmes, T. and Holdernesse, W. B., 'On the treatment of wounds by the application of carbolic acid, on Lister's method', *St. George's Hospital Reports*, 3, 1868.

Howie, W. B., 'The administration of an eighteenth century provincial hospital', *Medical History*, January, 1961.

Hussey, E. L., 'Statistical report of cases of amputation, lithotomy, and hernia, in the Radcliffe Infirmary, Oxford', *Transactions of the Provincial Medical and Surgical Association*, 7 (new series), 1853.

Hussey, E. L., 'Analysis of cases of amputation of the limbs in the Radcliffe Infirmary, Oxford', *Medico-Chirurgical Transactions*, 39, 1856.

James, J. H., 'On the causes of death after amputations of the limbs', *Transactions of the Provincial Medical and Surgical Association*, 17, 1850.

James, J. H., 'On the causes of mortality, after amputation of the limbs, part 2', *Transactions of the Provincial Medical and Surgical Association*, 18, 1851.

Johnson, J. G., 'A report of the surgical patients admitted into the Norfolk and Norwich Hospital, 1st January to 31st December 1834', *Transactions of the Provincial Medical and Surgical Association*, 4, 1836.

Jones, T., 'On the recent outbreak of small-pox at St. George's Hospital', *St. George's Hospital Reports*, 5, 1870.

Knight, A., 'On the grinders' asthma', *North of England Medical and Surgical Journal*, 1, 1830.

Langford, A. W., 'The history of Hereford General Hospital', *Transactions of the Woolhope Naturalists Field Club*, 1959.

Lawrie, J. A., 'On the results of amputations', *London Medical Gazette*, 1 (new series), 1841.

Lee, R., 'An analysis of 108 cases of ovariotomy which have occurred in Great Britain', *Medico-Chirurgical Transactions*, 34, 1851.

Leicester, H. A., 'Worcester General Infirmary – short history', *Berrow's Worcester Journal*, 14 October 1913.

Lyon, E., 'Sketch of the medical statistics and topography of Manchester', *North of England Medical and Surgical Journal*, 1, 1830.

McKeown, T. and Brown, R. G., 'Medical evidence related to English population changes in the eighteenth century', *Population Studies*, 9, 1955–6.

Martineau, P. M., 'On lithotomy', *Medico-Chirurgical Transactions*, 9, 1821.

Mouat, F. J., 'The president's address', *Journal of the Royal Statistical Society*, 1890.

Nunneley, T., 'Address in surgery', *British Medical Journal*, 7 August 1869.

Phillips, B., 'Mortality of amputation', *Journal of the Statistical Society*, June 1838.

Potter, J. P., 'Results of amputations at University College Hospital, London, statistically arranged', *Medico-Chirurgical Transactions*, 24, 1841.

Rabenn, W. B., 'Hospital diets in eighteenth century England', *Journal of the American Dietetic Association*, 30, 1954.

Razzell, P. E., 'Population change in eighteenth-century England: a re-appraisal', *Economic History Review*, 18, 2nd series, 1965.

Richardson, B. W., 'The medical history of England', *Medical Times and Gazette*, 1860–4.

Richmond, P. A., 'Glossary of historical fever terminology', *Journal of the History of Medicine*, 16, 1961.

Rook, A., 'Medical education and the English universities before 1800', *Journal of Medical Education*, 38, 1963.

Rosenberg, A., 'The London Dispensary for the Sick Poor', *Journal of the History of Medicine*, 14, 1959.

Sandwith, F. M., 'The nursing and care of the sick poor prior to 1850', *Hospital*, 1914.

Sigsworth, E. M., 'A provincial hospital in the eighteenth and early nineteenth centuries', *The College of General Practitioners, Yorkshire Faculty Journal*, 1966.

Simpson, J. Y., 'Hospitalism and its effects', *Edinburgh Medical Journal*, March and June 1869.

Smith, R., 'A statistical inquiry into the frequency of stone in the bladder in Great Britain and Ireland', *Medico-Chirurgical Transactions*, 11, 1820.

Statistical Society, 'Report of the Committee on Hospital Statistics', *Journal of the Statistical Society*, July 1842.

Statistical Society, 'Second Report of the Committee of the Statistical Society of London on Hospital Statistics', *Journal of the Statistical Society*, September 1844.

Statistical Society, 'Statistics of the general hospitals of London, 1861', *Journal of the Statistical Society*, 23 September 1862.

Statistical Society, 'Statistics of metropolitan and provincial general hospitals for 1862', *Journal of the Statistical Society*, 27 September 1864.

Statistical Society, 'Statistics of metropolitan and provincial general hospitals for 1863', *Journal of the Statistical Society*, 28 December 1865.

Statistical Society, 'Statistics of metropolitan and provincial general hospitals for 1864', *Journal of the Statistical Society*, 29 March 1866.

Steele, J. C., 'Numerical analysis of the patients treated in Guy's Hospital for the last seven years, from 1854 to 1861', *Journal of the Statistical Society*, 24, 1861.

Steele, J. C., 'The mortality of hospitals, general and special, in the United Kingdom, in times past and present', *Journal of the Statistical Society*, 40, 1877.

Steele, J. C., 'The charitable aspects of medical relief', *Journal of the Royal Statistical Society*, June 1891.

Stuart-Clark, A. C., 'Early hospital history – the later middle ages and the Tudors', *Hospital*, 55, 1959.

Thomson, S. C., 'The Great Windmill Street School', *Bulletin of the History of Medicine*, 12, 1942.

Underwood, E. A., 'Dumfries and the early history of surgical anaesthesia', *Annals of Science*, 23, 1967.

Waddy, F. F., 'The early history of Northampton General Hospital', *Northampton General Hospital Clinical Reports*, 1964.

Walker, J. K., 'Statistical observations on the medical charities of England and Ireland', *Transactions of the Provincial Medical and Surgical Association*, 4, 1836.

Walker, W. B., 'Medical education in 19th century Great Britain', *Journal of Medical Education*, 31, 1956.

Woodward, J. H., 'Before bacteriology: deaths in hospitals', *Royal College of General Practitioners, Yorkshire Faculty Journal*, autumn 1969.

Zimmerman, L. M., 'Surgeons and the rise of clinical teaching in England', *Bulletin of the History of Medicine*, 37, 1963.

Parliamentary Papers

Report of the Charity Commissioners – 1837.
Sixth Report of the Medical Officer of the Privy Council, 1863; Appendix 15, J. S. Bristowe and T. Holmes, *The Hospitals of the United Kingdom.*
Ninth Annual Report, Local Government Board, 1879–80.
Third Report, Select Committee on Metropolitan Hospitals, 1890–93.

Index

International Library of Sociology

Edited by
John Rex
University of Warwick

Founded by
Karl Mannheim
as The International Library of Sociology
and Social Reconstruction

*This Catalogue also contains other Social Science
series published by Routledge*

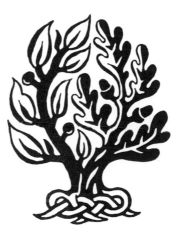

Routledge & Kegan Paul   London and Boston

68-74 Carter Lane London EC4V 5EL
9 Park Street Boston Mass 02108

Contents

● *Books so marked are available in paperback*
All books are in Metric Demy 8vo format (216 × 138mm approx.)

GENERAL SOCIOLOGY

Belshaw, Cyril. The Conditions of Social Performance. *An Exploratory Theory. 144 pp.*

Brown, Robert. Explanation in Social Science. *208 pp.*

● Rules and Laws in Sociology.

Cain, Maureen E. Society and the Policeman's Role. *About 300 pp.*

Gibson, Quentin. The Logic of Social Enquiry. *240 pp.*

Gurvitch, Georges. Sociology of Law. *Preface by Roscoe Pound. 264 pp.*

Homans, George C. Sentiments and Activities: *Essays in Social Science. 336 pp.*

Johnson, Harry M. Sociology: *a Systematic Introduction. Foreword by Robert K. Merton. 710 pp.*

Mannheim, Karl. Essays on Sociology and Social Psychology. *Edited by Paul Keckskemeti. With Editorial Note by Adolph Lowe. 344 pp.*

Systematic Sociology: *An Introduction to the Study of Society. Edited by J. S. Erös and Professor W. A. C. Stewart. 220 pp.*

Martindale, Don. The Nature and Types of Sociological Theory. *292 pp.*

● **Maus, Heinz.** A Short History of Sociology. *234 pp.*

Mey, Harald. Field-Theory. *A Study of its Application in the Social Sciences. 352 pp.*

Myrdal, Gunnar. Value in Social Theory: *A Collection of Essays on Methodology. Edited by Paul Streeten. 332 pp.*

Ogburn, William F., and **Nimkoff, Meyer F.** A Handbook of Sociology. *Preface by Karl Mannheim. 656 pp. 46 figures. 35 tables.*

Parsons, Talcott, and **Smelser, Neil J.** Economy and Society: *A Study in the Integration of Economic and Social Theory. 362 pp.*

● **Rex, John.** Key Problems of Sociological Theory. *220 pp.*

Urry, John. Reference Groups and the Theory of Revolution.

FOREIGN CLASSICS OF SOCIOLOGY

● **Durkheim, Emile.** Suicide. *A Study in Sociology. Edited and with an Introduction by George Simpson. 404 pp.*

Professional Ethics and Civic Morals. *Translated by Cornelia Brookfield. 288 pp.*

● **Gerth, H. H.,** and **Mills, C. Wright.** From Max Weber: *Essays in Sociology. 502 pp.*

Tönnies, Ferdinand. Community and Association. *(Gemeinschaft und Gesellschaft.) Translated and Supplemented by Charles P. Loomis. Foreword by Pitirim A. Sorokin. 334 pp.*

SOCIAL STRUCTURE

Andreski, Stanislav. Military Organization and Society. *Foreword by Professor A. R. Radcliffe-Brown. 226 pp. 1 folder.*

Coontz, Sydney H. Population Theories and the Economic Interpretation. *202 pp.*

Coser, Lewis. The Functions of Social Conflict. *204 pp.*

Dickie-Clark, H. F. Marginal Situation: *A Sociological Study of a Coloured Group. 240 pp. 11 tables.*

Glass, D. V. (Ed.). Social Mobility in Britain. *Contributions by J. Berent, T. Bottomore, R. C. Chambers, J. Floud, D. V. Glass, J. R. Hall, H. T. Himmelweit, R. K. Kelsall, F. M. Martin, C. A. Moser, R. Mukherjee, and W. Ziegel. 420 pp.*

Glaser, Barney, and **Strauss, Anselm L.** Status Passage. *A Formal Theory. 208 pp.*

Jones, Garth N. Planned Organizational Change: *An Exploratory Study Using an Empirical Approach. 268 pp.*

Kelsall, R. K. Higher Civil Servants in Britain: *From 1870 to the Present Day. 268 pp. 31 tables.*

König, René. The Community. *232 pp. Illustrated.*

● **Lawton, Denis.** Social Class, Language and Education. *192 pp.*

McLeish, John. The Theory of Social Change: *Four Views Considered. 128 pp.*

Marsh, David C. The Changing Social Structure of England and Wales, 1871-1961. *288 pp.*

Mouzelis, Nicos. Organization and Bureaucracy. *An Analysis of Modern Theories. 240 pp.*

Mulkay, M. J. Functionalism, Exchange and Theoretical Strategy. *272 pp.*

Ossowski, Stanislaw. Class Structure in the Social Consciousness. *210 pp.*

SOCIOLOGY AND POLITICS

Hertz, Frederick. Nationality in History and Politics: *A Psychology and Sociology of National Sentiment and Nationalism. 432 pp.*

Kornhauser, William. The Politics of Mass Society. *272 pp. 20 tables.*

Laidler, Harry W. History of Socialism. *Social-Economic Movements: An Historical and Comparative Survey of Socialism, Communism, Co-operation, Utopianism; and other Systems of Reform and Reconstruction. 992 pp.*

Mannheim, Karl. Freedom, Power and Democratic Planning. *Edited by Hans Gerth and Ernest K. Bramstedt. 424 pp.*

Mansur, Fatma. Process of Independence. *Foreword by A. H. Hanson. 208 pp.*

Martin, David A. Pacificism: *an Historical and Sociological Study. 262 pp.*

Myrdal, Gunnar. The Political Element in the Development of Economic Theory. *Translated from the German by Paul Streeten. 282 pp.*

Wootton, Graham. Workers, Unions and the State. *188 pp.*

FOREIGN AFFAIRS: THEIR SOCIAL, POLITICAL AND ECONOMIC FOUNDATIONS

Mayer, J. P. Political Thought in France from the Revolution to the Fifth Republic. *164 pp.*

CRIMINOLOGY

Ancel, Marc. Social Defence: *A Modern Approach to Criminal Problems.* *Foreword by Leon Radzinowicz. 240 pp.*

Cloward, Richard A., and **Ohlin, Lloyd E.** Delinquency and Opportunity: *A Theory of Delinquent Gangs. 248 pp.*

Downes, David M. The Delinquent Solution. *A Study in Subcultural Theory. 296 pp.*

Dunlop, A. B., and **McCabe, S.** Young Men in Detention Centres. *192 pp.*

Friedlander, Kate. The Psycho-Analytical Approach to Juvenile Delinquency: *Theory, Case Studies, Treatment. 320 pp.*

Glueck, Sheldon, and **Eleanor.** Family Environment and Delinquency. *With the statistical assistance of Rose W. Kneznek. 340 pp.*

Lopez-Rey, Manuel. Crime. *An Analytical Appraisal. 288 pp.*

Mannheim, Hermann. Comparative Criminology: *a Text Book. Two volumes. 442 pp. and 380 pp.*

Morris, Terence. The Criminal Area: *A Study in Social Ecology. Foreword by Hermann Mannheim. 232 pp. 25 tables. 4 maps.*

● **Taylor, Ian, Walton, Paul,** and **Young, Jock.** The New Criminology. *For a Social Theory of Deviance.*

SOCIAL PSYCHOLOGY

Bagley, Christopher. The Social Psychology of the Epileptic Child. *320 pp.*

Barbu, Zevedei. Problems of Historical Psychology. *248 pp.*

Blackburn, Julian. Psychology and the Social Pattern. *184 pp.*

● **Brittan, Arthur.** Meanings and Situations. *224 pp.*

● **Fleming, C. M.** Adolescence: Its Social Psychology. *With an Introduction to recent findings from the fields of Anthropology, Physiology, Medicine, Psychometrics and Sociometry. 288 pp.*

● The Social Psychology of Education: *An Introduction and Guide to Its Study. 136 pp.*

Homans, George C. The Human Group. *Foreword by Bernard DeVoto. Introduction by Robert K. Merton. 526 pp.*

Social Behaviour: *its Elementary Forms. 416 pp.*

Klein, Josephine. The Study of Groups. *226 pp. 31 figures. 5 tables.*

Linton, Ralph. The Cultural Background of Personality. *132 pp.*

Mayo, Elton. The Social Problems of an Industrial Civilization. *With an appendix on the Political Problem. 180 pp.*

Ottaway, A. K. C. Learning Through Group Experience. *176 pp.*

Ridder, J. C. de. The Personality of the Urban African in South Africa. *A Thematic Apperception Test Study. 196 pp. 12 plates.*

● **Rose, Arnold M.** (Ed.). Human Behaviour and Social Processes: *an Interactionist Approach. Contributions by Arnold M. Rose, Ralph H. Turner, Anselm Strauss, Everett C. Hughes, E. Franklin Frazier, Howard S. Becker, et al. 696 pp.*

Smelser, Neil J. Theory of Collective Behaviour. *448 pp.*
Stephenson, Geoffrey M. The Development of Conscience. *128 pp.*
Young, Kimball. Handbook of Social Psychology. *658 pp. 16 figures. 10 tables.*

SOCIOLOGY OF THE FAMILY

Banks, J. A. Prosperity and Parenthood: *A Study of Family Planning among The Victorian Middle Classes. 262 pp.*
Bell, Colin R. Middle Class Families: *Social and Geographical Mobility. 224 pp.*
Burton, Lindy. Vulnerable Children. *272 pp.*
Gavron, Hannah. The Captive Wife: *Conflicts of Household Mothers. 190 pp.*
George, Victor, and **Wilding, Paul.** Motherless Families. *220 pp.*
Klein, Josephine. Samples from English Cultures.
 1. Three Preliminary Studies and Aspects of Adult Life in England. *447 pp.*
 2. Child-Rearing Practices and Index. *247 pp.*
Klein, Viola. Britain's Married Women Workers. *180 pp.*
 The Feminine Character. *History of an Ideology. 244 pp.*
McWhinnie, Alexina M. Adopted Children. *How They Grow Up. 304 pp.*
Myrdal, Alva, and **Klein, Viola.** Women's Two Roles: *Home and Work. 238 pp. 27 tables.*
Parsons, Talcott, and **Bales, Robert F.** Family: Socialization and Interaction Process. *In collaboration with James Olds, Morris Zelditch and Philip E. Slater. 456 pp. 50 figures and tables.*

SOCIAL SERVICES

Bastide, Roger. The Sociology of Mental Disorder. *Translated from the French by Jean McNeil. 260 pp.*
Carlebach, Julius. Caring For Children in Trouble. *266 pp.*
Forder, R. A. (Ed.). Penelope Hall's Social Services of England and Wales. *352 pp.*
George, Victor. Foster Care. *Theory and Practice. 234 pp.*
 Social Security: *Beveridge and After. 258 pp.*
● **Goetschius, George W.** Working with Community Groups. *256 pp.*
Goetschius, George W., and **Tash, Joan.** Working with Unattached Youth. *416 pp.*
Hall, M. P., and **Howes, I. V.** The Church in Social Work. *A Study of Moral Welfare Work undertaken by the Church of England. 320 pp.*
Heywood, Jean S. Children in Care: *the Development of the Service for the Deprived Child. 264 pp.*
Hoenig, J., and **Hamilton, Marian W.** The De-Segration of the Mentally Ill. *284 pp.*
Jones, Kathleen. Mental Health and Social Policy, 1845-1959. *264 pp.*

King, Roy D., Raynes, Norma V., and **Tizard, Jack.** Patterns of Residential Care. *356 pp.*

Leigh, John. Young People and Leisure. *256 pp.*

Morris, Mary. Voluntary Work and the Welfare State. *300 pp.*

Morris, Pauline. Put Away: *A Sociological Study of Institutions for the Mentally Retarded. 364 pp.*

Nokes, P. L. The Professional Task in Welfare Practice. *152 pp.*

Timms, Noel. Psychiatric Social Work in Great Britain (1939-1962). *280 pp.*

● Social Casework: *Principles and Practice. 256 pp.*

Young, A. F., and **Ashton, E. T.** British Social Work in the Nineteenth Century. *288 pp.*

Young, A. F. Social Services in British Industry. *272 pp.*

SOCIOLOGY OF EDUCATION

Banks, Olive. Parity and Prestige in English Secondary Education: a Study in Educational Sociology. *272 pp.*

Bentwich, Joseph. Education in Israel. *224 pp. 8 pp. plates.*

● **Blyth, W. A. L.** English Primary Education. *A Sociological Description.*
　1. Schools. *232 pp.*
　2. Background. *168 pp.*

Collier, K. G. The Social Purposes of Education: *Personal and Social Values in Education. 268 pp.*

Dale, R. R., and **Griffith, S.** Down Stream: *Failure in the Grammar School. 108 pp.*

Dore, R. P. Education in Tokugawa Japan. *356 pp. 9 pp. plates*

Evans, K. M. Sociometry and Education. *158 pp.*

Foster, P. J. Education and Social Change in Ghana. *336 pp. 3 maps.*

Fraser, W. R. Education and Society in Modern France. *150 pp.*

Grace, Gerald R. Role Conflict and the Teacher. *About 200 pp.*

Hans, Nicholas. New Trends in Education in the Eighteenth Century. *278 pp. 19 tables.*

● Comparative Education: *A Study of Educational Factors and Traditions. 360 pp.*

Hargreaves, David. Interpersonal Relations and Education. *432 pp.*

● Social Relations in a Secondary School. *240 pp.*

Holmes, Brian. Problems in Education. *A Comparative Approach. 336 pp.*

King, Ronald. Values and Involvement in a Grammar School. *164 pp.*
School Organization and Pupil Involvement. *A Study of Secondary Schools.*

● **Mannheim, Karl,** and **Stewart, W. A. C.** An Introduction to the Sociology of Education. *206 pp.*

Morris, Raymond N. The Sixth Form and College Entrance. *231 pp.*

● **Musgrove, F.** Youth and the Social Order. *176 pp.*

● **Ottaway, A. K. C.** Education and Society: An Introduction to the Sociology of Education. *With an Introduction by W. O. Lester Smith. 212 pp.*

Peers, Robert. Adult Education: *A Comparative Study. 398 pp.*

7

Pritchard, D. G. Education and the Handicapped: *1760 to 1960. 258 pp.*
Richardson, Helen. Adolescent Girls in Approved Schools. *308 pp.*
Stratta, Erica. The Education of Borstal Boys. *A Study of their Educational Experiences prior to, and during Borstal Training. 256 pp.*

SOCIOLOGY OF CULTURE

Eppel, E. M., and **M.** Adolescents and Morality: *A Study of some Moral Values and Dilemmas of Working Adolescents in the Context of a changing Climate of Opinion. Foreword by W. J. H. Sprott. 268 pp. 39 tables.*
● **Fromm, Erich.** The Fear of Freedom. *286 pp.*
The Sane Society. *400 pp.*
Mannheim, Karl. Essays on the Sociology of Culture. *Edited by Ernst Mannheim in co-operation with Paul Kecskemeti. Editorial Note by Adolph Lowe. 280 pp.*
Weber, Alfred. Farewell to European History: *or The Conquest of Nihilism Translated from the German by R. F. C. Hull. 224 pp.*

SOCIOLOGY OF RELIGION

Argyle, Michael. Religious Behaviour. *224 pp. 8 figures. 41 tables.*
Nelson, G. K. Spiritualism and Society. *313 pp.*
Stark, Werner. The Sociology of Religion. *A Study of Christendom.*
Volume I. *Established Religion. 248 pp.*
Volume II. *Sectarian Religion. 368 pp.*
Volume III. *The Universal Church. 464 pp.*
Volume IV. *Types of Religious Man. 352 pp.*
Volume V. *Types of Religious Culture. 464 pp.*
Watt, W. Montgomery. Islam and the Integration of Society. *320 pp.*

SOCIOLOGY OF ART AND LITERATURE

Jarvie, Ian C. Towards a Sociology of the Cinema. *A Comparative Essay on the Structure and Functioning of a Major Entertainment Industry. 405 pp.*
Rust, Frances S. Dance in Society. *An Analysis of the Relationships between the Social Dance and Society in England from the Middle Ages to the Present Day. 256 pp. 8 pp. of plates.*
Schücking, L. L. The Sociology of Literary Taste. *112 pp.*

SOCIOLOGY OF KNOWLEDGE

Mannheim, Karl. Essays on the Sociology of Knowledge. *Edited by Paul Kecskemeti. Editorial Note by Adolph Lowe. 353 pp.*

Remmling, Gunter W. (Ed.). Towards the Sociology of Knowledge. *Origins and Development of a Sociological Thought Style.*

Stark, Werner. The Sociology of Knowledge: *An Essay in Aid of a Deeper Understanding of the History of Ideas. 384 pp.*

URBAN SOCIOLOGY

Ashworth, William. The Genesis of Modern British Town Planning: *A Study in Economic and Social History of the Nineteenth and Twentieth Centuries. 288 pp.*

Cullingworth, J. B. Housing Needs and Planning Policy: *A Restatement of the Problems of Housing Need and 'Overspill' in England and Wales. 232 pp. 44 tables. 8 maps.*

Dickinson, Robert E. City and Region: *A Geographical Interpretation. 608 pp. 125 figures.*

The West European City: *A Geographical Interpretation. 600 pp. 129 maps. 29 plates.*

● The City Region in Western Europe. *320 pp. Maps.*

Humphreys, Alexander J. New Dubliners: *Urbanization and the Irish Family. Foreword by George C. Homans. 304 pp.*

Jackson, Brian. Working Class Community: *Some General Notions raised by a Series of Studies in Northern England. 192 pp.*

Jennings, Hilda. Societies in the Making: *a Study of Development and Re-development within a County Borough. Foreword by D. A. Clark. 286 pp.*

● **Mann, P. H.** An Approach to Urban Sociology. *240 pp.*

Morris, R. N., and **Mogey, J.** The Sociology of Housing. *Studies at Berinsfield. 232 pp. 4 pp. plates.*

Rosser, C., and **Harris, C.** The Family and Social Change. *A Study of Family and Kinship in a South Wales Town. 352 pp. 8 maps.*

RURAL SOCIOLOGY

Chambers, R. J. H. Settlement Schemes in Tropical Africa: *A Selective Study. 268 pp.*

Haswell, M. R. The Economics of Development in Village India. *120 pp.*

Littlejohn, James. Westrigg: *the Sociology of a Cheviot Parish. 172 pp. 5 figures.*

Mayer, Adrian C. Peasants in the Pacific. *A Study of Fiji Indian Rural Society. 248 pp. 20 plates.*

Williams, W. M. The Sociology of an English Village: *Gosforth. 272 pp. 12 figures. 13 tables.*

SOCIOLOGY OF INDUSTRY AND DISTRIBUTION

Anderson, Nels. Work and Leisure. *280 pp.*

● **Blau, Peter M.**, and **Scott, W. Richard.** Formal Organizations: *a Comparative approach. Introduction and Additional Bibliography by J. H. Smith. 326 pp.*

Eldridge, J. E. T. Industrial Disputes. *Essays in the Sociology of Industrial Relations. 288 pp.*

Hetzler, Stanley. Applied Measures for Promoting Technological Growth. *352 pp.*

Technological Growth and Social Change. *Achieving Modernization. 269 pp.*

Hollowell, Peter G. The Lorry Driver. *272 pp.*

Jefferys, Margot, *with the assistance of Winifred Moss.* Mobility in the Labour Market: *Employment Changes in Battersea and Dagenham. Preface by Barbara Wootton. 186 pp. 51 tables.*

Millerson, Geoffrey. The Qualifying Associations: *a Study in Professionalization. 320 pp.*

Smelser, Neil J. Social Change in the Industrial Revolution: *An Application of Theory to the Lancashire Cotton Industry, 1770-1840. 468 pp. 12 figures. 14 tables.*

Williams, Gertrude. Recruitment to Skilled Trades. *240 pp.*

Young, A. F. Industrial Injuries Insurance: *an Examination of British Policy. 192 pp.*

DOCUMENTARY

Schlesinger, Rudolf (Ed.). Changing Attitudes in Soviet Russia.
   2. The Nationalities Problem and Soviet Administration. *Selected Readings on the Development of Soviet Nationalities Policies. Introduced by the editor. Translated by W. W. Gottlieb. 324 pp.*

ANTHROPOLOGY

Ammar, Hamed. Growing up in an Egyptian Village: *Silwa, Province of Aswan. 336 pp.*

Brandel-Syrier, Mia. Reeftown Elite. *A Study of Social Mobility in a Modern African Community on the Reef. 376 pp.*

Crook, David, and **Isabel.** Revolution in a Chinese Village: *Ten Mile Inn. 230 pp. 8 plates. 1 map.*

Dickie-Clark, H. F. The Marginal Situation. *A Sociological Study of a Coloured Group. 236 pp.*

Dube, S. C. Indian Village. *Foreword by Morris Edward Opler. 276 pp. 4 plates.*

India's Changing Villages: *Human Factors in Community Development. 260 pp. 8 plates. 1 map.*

Firth, Raymond. Malay Fishermen. *Their Peasant Economy. 420 pp. 17 pp. plates.*

Gulliver, P. H. Social Control in an African Society: a Study of the Arusha, Agricultural Masai of Northern Tanganyika. *320 pp. 8 plates. 10 figures.*

Ishwaran, K. Shivapur. *A South Indian Village. 216 pp.*
Tradition and Economy in Village India: *An Interactionist Approach. Foreword by Conrad Arensburg. 176 pp.*

Jarvie, Ian C. The Revolution in Anthropology. *268 pp.*

Jarvie, Ian C., and **Agassi, Joseph.** Hong Kong. *A Society in Transition. 396 pp. Illustrated with plates and maps.*

Little, Kenneth L. Mende of Sierra Leone. *308 pp. and folder.*
Negroes in Britain. *With a New Introduction and Contemporary Study by Leonard Bloom. 320 pp.*

Lowie, Robert H. Social Organization. *494 pp.*

Mayer, Adrian C. Caste and Kinship in Central India: *A Village and its Region. 328 pp. 16 plates. 15 figures. 16 tables.*

Smith, Raymond T. The Negro Family in British Guiana: *Family Structure and Social Status in the Villages. With a Foreword by Meyer Fortes. 314 pp. 8 plates. 1 figure. 4 maps.*

SOCIOLOGY AND PHILOSOPHY

Barnsley, John H. The Social Reality of Ethics. *A Comparative Analysis of Moral Codes. 448 pp.*

Diesing, Paul. Patterns of Discovery in the Social Sciences. *362 pp.*

Douglas, Jack D. (Ed.). Understanding Everyday Life. *Toward the Reconstruction of Sociological Knowledge. Contributions by Alan F. Blum. Aaron W. Cicourel, Norman K. Denzin, Jack D. Douglas, John Heeren, Peter McHugh, Peter K. Manning, Melvin Power, Matthew Speier, Roy Turner, D. Lawrence Wieder, Thomas P. Wilson and Don H. Zimmerman. 370 pp.*

Jarvie, Ian C. Concepts and Society. *216 pp.*

Roche, Maurice. Phenomenology, Language and the Social Sciences. *About 400 pp.*

Sahay, Arun. Sociological Analysis.

Sklair, Leslie. The Sociology of Progress. *320 pp.*

International Library of Anthropology

General Editor Adam Kuper

Brown, Paula. The Chimbu. *A Study of Change in the New Guinea Highlands.*
Van Den Berghe, Pierre L. Power and Privilege at an African University.

International Library
of Social Policy
General Editor Kathleen Jones

Holman, Robert. Trading in Children. *A Study of Private Fostering.*
Jones, Kathleen. History of the Mental Health Services. *428 pp.*
Thomas, J. E. The English Prison Officer since 1850: *A Study in Conflict.*
258 pp.

Primary Socialization, Language
and Education
General Editor Basil Bernstein

Bernstein, Basil. Class, Codes and Control. *2 volumes.*
  1. *Theoretical Studies Towards a Sociology of Language. 254 pp.*
  2. *Applied Studies Towards a Sociology of Language. About 400 pp.*
Brandis, Walter, and **Henderson, Dorothy.** Social Class, Language and
  Communication. *288 pp.*
Cook-Gumperz, Jenny. Social Control and Socialization. *A Study of Class
  Differences in the Language of Maternal Control.*
Gahagan, D. M., and **G. A.** Talk Reform. *Exploration in Language for Infant
  School Children. 160 pp.*
Robinson, W. P., and **Rackstraw, Susan, D. A.** A Question of Answers.
  2 volumes. 192 pp. and 180 pp.
Turner, Geoffrey, J., and **Mohan, Bernard, A.** A Linguistic Description and
  Computer Programme for Children's Speech. *208 pp.*

Reports of the Institute of Community Studies

Cartwright, Ann. Human Relations and Hospital Care. *272 pp.*
  Parents and Family Planning Services. *306 pp.*
  Patients and their Doctors. *A Study of General Practice. 304 pp.*
● **Jackson, Brian.** Streaming: *an Education System in Miniature. 168 pp.*
Jackson, Brian, and **Marsden, Dennis.** Education and the Working Class:
  *Some General Themes raised by a Study of 88 Working-class Children
  in a Northern Industrial City. 268 pp. 2 folders.*
Marris, Peter. The Experience of Higher Education. *232 pp. 27 tables.*
Marris, Peter, and **Rein, Martin.** Dilemmas of Social Reform. *Poverty and
  Community Action in the United States. 256 pp.*
Marris, Peter, and **Somerset, Anthony.** African Businessmen. *A Study of
  Entrepreneurship and Development in Kenya. 256 pp.*
Mills, Richard. Young Outsiders: *a Study in Alternative Communities.*